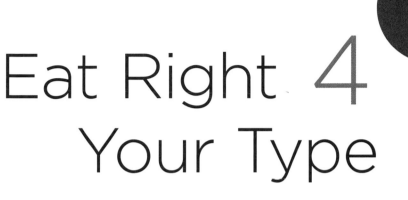

TYPE
O

Eat Right 4
Your Type

PERSONALIZED COOKBOOK

TYPE O

Eat Right 4 Your Type

PERSONALIZED COOKBOOK

150+ Healthy Recipes for Your Blood Type Diet®

Dr. Peter J. D'Adamo
with Kristin O'Connor

Photographs by Kristin O'Connor

Previously published as *Personalized Living Using the Blood Type Diet® (Type O)*

B

BERKLEY BOOKS, NEW YORK

THE BERKLEY PUBLISHING GROUP

Published by the Penguin Group

Penguin Group (USA) LLC

375 Hudson Street, New York, New York 10014, USA

USA | Canada | UK | Ireland | Australia | New Zealand | India | South Africa | China

Penguin Books Ltd., Registered Offices: 80 Strand, London WC2R 0RL, England

For more information about the Penguin Group, visit penguin.com.

Library of Congress Cataloging-in-Publication Data

D'Adamo, Peter J.
Eat right 4 your type personalized cookbook type O : 150+ healthy recipes for your blood type diet / Dr. Peter J. D'Adamo with Kristin O'Connor; photographs by Kristin O'Connor.
    p. cm.
  ISBN 978-0-425-26948-0 (pbk.)
  1. Diet therapy. 2. Nutrition. 3. Blood groups. 4. Naturopathy. I. O'Connor, Kristin. II. Title. III. Title: Eat right for your type personalized cookbook type O.
  RM219.D292 2013
  641.5'631—dc23
                          2013021051

PUBLISHING HISTORY

Previously published in eBook format as *Personalized Living Using the Blood Type Diet®* *(Type O)* by Drum Hill Publishing, LLC in 2012
Berkley trade paperback edition / October 2013

PRINTED IN THE UNITED STATES OF AMERICA

10   9   8   7   6

Cover design by Jason Gill
Cover photo by Christopher Bierlein
Book design by Pauline Neuwirth

Contents

Introduction   1

Type O at a Glance   5

First Things First   7

Breakfast   23

    Quinoa Muesli   24

    Blackstrap-Cherry Granola NS   25

    Granola–Nut Butter Fruit Slices   26

    Breakfast Egg Salad   27

    Turkey Bacon–Spinach Squares   29

    Swiss Chard and Cremini Frittata NS   30

    Broccoli-Feta Frittata   31

    Maple-Sausage Scramble   33

    Homemade Turkey Breakfast Sausage   34

    Savory Herb and Cheese Bread Pudding   35

    Spinach-Zucchini Soufflé   36

    Cinnamon-Millet Crêpes   37

    Brown Rice Pancakes   39

    Wild-Rice Waffles   41

    Pumpkin Muffins with Carob Drizzle   42

    Pear-Rosemary Bread NS   43

    Cherry Scones   44

 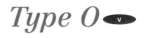

Blueberry-Macadamia Muffins   46

Lunch   47

Adzuki Hummus Sandwich NS   48

Bacon Grilled Cheese   48

Lamb Meatball Subs NS   49

Philly Cheesesteak Sandwich   51

Greens and Beans Salad NS   52

Salad Pizza   53

*Dandelion Greens with Roasted Roots
    and Horseradish Dressing* NS   55

Roasted Tomato Greek Salad   56

Salmon-Salad Radicchio Cups   57

Baked Falafel NS   58

Raw Kale Salad with Zesty Lime Dressing NS   59

Crunchy Kohlrabi Spring Rolls with Sweet Cherry Dip NS   60

Feta, Spinach, and Asparagus Pie   62

Ratatouille NS   65

White Bean Stew NS   66

Dinner   67

Roasted Tomato and Broccoli Mac and Cheese   68

Pasta Carbonara with Crispy Kale   69

Spring Pesto Pasta   71

Sweet Potato Gnocchi with Basil-Cranberry Sauce NS   73

Veggie Lasagna   74

Grilled Radicchio and Walnut-Spinach Pesto NS   76

Noodles with Poached Salmon and Creamy Basil Sauce NS   77

Salmon–Black Bean Cakes with Creamy Cilantro Sauce NS   78

Lemon-Ginger Salmon   79

Baked Mahimahi with Crunchy Fennel Salad   80

Parchment-Baked Snapper NS   81

Fig and Basil Halibut NS   83

Spicy Seafood Stew NS   84

Fish Tacos with Sweet Mango-Bean Salad   87

Seafood Paella   89

Fig-Stuffed Turkey Breasts NS   91

Turkey Sausage–Stuffed Peppers NS   93

Turkey-Ginger Stir-Fry NS   94

Hearty Slow-Cooker Turkey Stew NS   95

Turkey Mole Drumsticks   97

Crispy-Coated Turkey Tenderloins with Apricot Dipping Sauce   99

Shredded Turkey Bake   100

Green Tea–Poached Chicken NS   101

Chicken Pot Pie with Crunchy Topping NS   103

Broccolini-Stuffed Chicken   104

Beef Tips with Wild Mushrooms NS   106

Beef and Bean Chili   107

Braised Brisket   109

Tangy Pineapple and Beef Kabobs NS   111

Sweet Potato Shepherd's Pie   112

Sun-Dried Tomato Burgers on Millet Buns NS   114

Grilled Lamb Chops with Mint Pesto NS   115

Moroccan Lamb Tagine   117

Slow-Cooker Venison NS   118

Meat Loaf   119

Red Quinoa–Mushroom Casserole with Fried Eggs NS   120

Sprouted Lentil Stew NS   123

Spaghetti Squash with Goat Cheese and Walnuts   124

Type O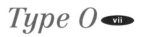

Soups and Sides

Soups and Sides   125

Thai Curry Soup NS   126

Carrot-Ginger Soup NS   127

Roasted Parsnip Soup   128

Melted Mozzarella–Onion Soup   129

Broccoli–Northern Bean Soup NS   130

Beef and Shredded Escarole Soup NS   131

Wild-Grain Soup with Sun-Dried Tomato Pesto NS   133

Tomato-Basil Soup NS   134

Sweet and Crunchy Kohlrabi Slaw NS   135

Sweet-and-Salty Brussels   137

Grilled Sesame-Ginger Bok Choy NS   138

South Indian–Curried Okra NS   139

Baked Beans NS   140

Spicy Collards NS   141

Garlic-Creamed Spinach   142

Roasted Escarole NS   143

Roasted Pumpkin with Fried Sage NS   145

Roasted Broccoli and Tomatoes NS   146

Sweet Potato Hash with Turkey Sausage   147

Autumn Roasted Roots NS   149

Rutabaga Smash   151

Whipped Sweet Potato Soufflé   152

Kohlrabi Gratin with Sage-Walnut Cream   153

Tomato and Broccoli Ragu NS   154

Creamy Rice Polenta   155

Brown Rice Salad NS   156

Forbidden Black Rice Risotto NS   157

Herbed Quinoa   158

Crisp-Tender Veggie Quinoa NS 159

Roasted Wakame and Fennel Salad NS 161

Mint and Cherry Tomato Tabbouleh NS 162

Snacks 163

Toasty Pizza Bites 164

Heirloom Tomato Salsa 165

Crudités and Creamy Goat Cheese Dip S *(S Only!)* 166

Adzuki Bean Hummus NS 167

Flax Crackers NS 169

Curried Egg Salad NS 171

Farmer Cheese and Beet-Endive Cups 172

Marinated Mozzarella S *(S Only!)* 173

Spicy Rosemary-Nut Mix 174

Crispy Spring Vegetable Cakes NS 175

Crispy Walnut Bacon–Wrapped Asparagus NS 177

Artichoke Bruschetta 179

Baked Grapefruit 180

Fruit Salad with Mint-Lime Dressing NS 181

Homemade Applesauce 182

Pear and Apple Chips 183

Grilled Pineapple with Cinnamon Syrup 184

Almond Butter Rice Cakes with Mini Chips 185

Carob–Walnut Butter–Stuffed Figs NS 186

Drinks and Beverages 187

Cooling Chamomile Spritzer NS 188

Cherry Spritzer NS 188

Carrot, Kale, and Ginger Juice 189

Sweet Basil and Ginger Tea NS 190

Type O 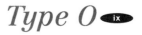 ix

Mango-Kale Smoothie 190

Matcha-Mojito Tea 191

Creamy Banana–Nut Butter Smoothie 193

Pineapple Spa Water NS 194

Berry Bonanza Smoothie 194

Desserts 195

Deep-Chocolate Brownies 197

Chocolate Salted-Nut Clusters NS 198

Chocolate Chip Cookies 199

Cocoa-Dusted Chocolate Truffles 201

Almond-Cranberry Biscotti 203

Fig Bars 205

Blueberry Crumble 206

Peach-Cinnamon Charlotte 207

Carrot-Pineapple Cake with Chocolate-Chai Frosting 208

Upside-Down Almond Cake with Apricot Glaze 209

Matcha Cake with Chocolate Frosting 211

Crêpes with Raspberry Chutney NS 212

Banana-Based Ice Cream: 4 Ways 214

Ginger-Rice Pudding 216

Stocks, Condiments, and Sauces 217

Ketchup Substitute 218

Herb Dressing NS 218

Carrot-Ginger Dressing NS 219

Chocolate Syrup NS 219

Cinnamon Syrup 220

Chicken or Turkey Stock NS 221

Beef Stock NS 222

Vegetable Stock NS   223

Basic Gluten-Free Bread Crumbs NS   224

USEFUL TOOLS   225

Menus   227

   Substitutions   227

   Menu Planning   229

   Four-Week Meal Planner   230

Tools   237

Food Journal   237

Tracking Your Progress   237

Shopping List   237

Time to Think Green   239

Quick Review of the Terms   239

Tips for Buying Local and Organic   240

Dirty Dozen/Clean Fifteen   242

Safe Food Storage   243

Cleaning up the Kitchen   245

Appendix I: Additional Information on the Blood Type Diet   247

Discover Your Blood Type   247

Secretor Status   247

Center of Excellence in Generative Medicine   247

D'Adamo Personalized Nutrition®—North American Pharmacal, Inc.   248

www.dadamo.com—For All Things Peter D'Adamo   248

Appendix II: Products   249

Protein Blend™ Powder—Type O   249

Unibar® Protein Bar   249

 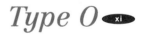

Carob Extract™   249

Proberry 3™ *Liquid*   250

SWAMI© Personalized Nutrition Software Program   250

Appendix III: References   251

Acknowledgments   253

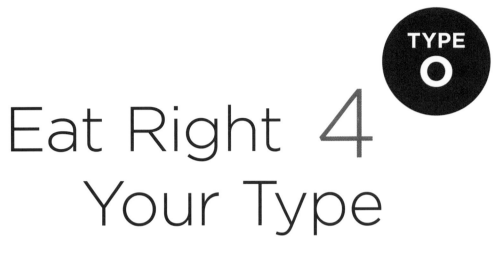

Eat Right 4 Your Type

PERSONALIZED COOKBOOK

Introduction

Let food be thy medicine,

and medicine be thy food.

—HIPPOCRATES

FOOD HAS THE potential to heal and strengthen our physical bodies, support our recovery from injury and illness, and potentially change our genetic destinies.

Not only does food provide sustenance and nourishment, it provides an opportunity for creative expression and community, whether through developing new recipes or ways to prepare a certain food or in sharing a meal with others. When I wrote *Eat Right 4 Your Type* in 1996, I explored the connections between blood type and diet, and outlined specific nutritional programs for each blood type. Since its publication more than fifteen years ago, I have continued to research and write about the role that foods play in our lives, and I have tried to create support materials and guidance for people who follow the Blood Type Diet.

In 1998, I wrote *Cook Right 4 Your Type*, which acted as a handbook for my readers, providing recipes, cooking tips, and planning guidelines to help navigate the process of food planning and preparation. I always wanted to take this further, as I felt there was an aesthetic quality about food and food preparation that should be reflected in a book, not just with great recipes but also with beautiful, four-color photography that celebrates food. About three years ago, I met Kristin O'Connor. Although she came to see me as a patient, our conversation turned to following the Blood Type Diet, cooking, food preparation, and the work she was doing as a personal chef, food stylist, and food blogger.

I was impressed by her dedication to nutrition and healthy eating, and with her ability to simplify the food-preparation process, which for some people can be quite daunting. Over the ensuing months, as we worked together as doctor and patient, our conversations returned again and again to food. I felt that I found in Kristin the perfect person to collaborate on a book project that would blend the scientific concepts of the Blood Type Diet with the artistry of cooking to create visually stunning cookbooks specifically designed for each blood type. Kristin has a passion for the Blood Type Diet that is unparalleled and an encyclopedic knowledge of the

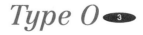

Type O **3**

food lists for each of the blood types. She is creative and resourceful, and she appreciates and respects the need for food to both taste delicious and be nourishing.

For the past year, I have been enjoying the recipes included in the books, and I have to say that I've been knocked out by how delicious they are. They are also easy to prepare, as I know most of us have limited hours in the day for food planning and preparation. The recipes contained in these books are suitable for individuals or families as well as for special events and entertaining. Additionally, there are helpful food preparation tips, suggestions for how to organize your kitchen, food storage guidelines, and suggested resources that can make meal planning and preparation easier. My goal has always been to provide accessible information that is easy to incorporate into daily life, and I believe that Kristin has accomplished this.

These cookbooks represent new food and healthy lifestyle possibilities for my readers; they combine the science behind the Blood Type Diet with Kristin's expertise as a chef and believer of these concepts, and package them in a beautiful, four-color format. The recipes contained within are appropriate for your blood type and compliant with the food lists, and they are delicious and made with love—love of food, love of health, and love of sharing this with others on both Kristin's and my part.

I invite you to join us on the continued journey of personalized living. I am confident that you will find a trusted companion in these cookbooks, one that will make your life richer and healthier as you experiment with the recipes that were developed specifically to be right for your type.

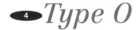

Type O at a Glance

MANY TYPE Os are thrilled to find that when they scan their lists of *Beneficial*, *Neutral*, and *Avoids*, both chocolate and beef are classified as *Beneficial*. You might be saying to yourself, "Am I really on a 'diet' where chocolate promotes weight loss?" The answer is "Yes." The difference is that *Eat Right 4 Your Type* is not a typical diet; it is a way of eating to create an optimal environment for health in your body. It is for this reason that this "diet" works on issues like weight loss simultaneously with disease prevention and reduction. The question now is, what does it mean to be on a Type O diet?

From a dietary perspective, those with Type O blood thrive on high-quality animal protein, limited grains, fruits, and vegetables. Among the type's major downfalls are wheat, corn, navy beans, lentils, kidney beans, and most dairy. But don't worry; following a wheat- and/or gluten-free diet no longer means having to sacrifice and live without bread. Wheat-free and gluten-free products are among the fastest growing items in the food world today, making it easier and easier to find pizza, breads, pastas, and flours so that you don't have to miss out on the things you love. Type Os thrive on a protein-rich diet and low amounts of grains for optimal health and weight-loss. Some mouth-watering *Beneficial* foods for Type O are lamb, beef, kale, broccoli, chocolate, green tea, pineapple, cherries, and bananas. This is just a small list of delicious foods that are also incredibly healing for the Type O body.

What are Type Os most likely to be healing from? Susceptibilities in Type Os typically present as ulcers and irritation resulting from high acidity in the stomach, as well as thyroid disorders often caused by insufficient levels of iodine, yeast overgrowth, gut inflammation, or deficiencies of the amino acid tyrosine. These problems can be corrected through the *Eat Right 4 Your Type* diet. For example, seaweed is a highly *Beneficial* food for Type O; it naturally contains iodine and can help improve thyroid function and metabolic rate. Therefore, when you are eating right for your blood type, you are compensating for any imbalances and optimizing your health's potential.

 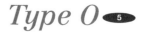

The Blood Type Diet has taken personalized nutrition to a higher level with the influence that Secretor Status has on our health. Approximately 80 percent of the population are Secretors, which means that the majority of us secrete our blood-type antigens through bodily fluids such as saliva and mucus. As I write about in *Live Right 4 Your Type*:

> Subtyping your blood, especially your Secretor Status, provides an even greater specificity of identification. Your blood type doesn't just sit inert in your body. It is expressed in countless ways . . . A simple analogy would be a faucet. Depending on the water pressure, the faucet might pour or dribble . . . In the same way, your Secretor Status relates to how much and where your blood type antigen is expressed in your body.

Being a Secretor means that the secretions in a person's saliva can immediately attack viruses, bacteria, and other foreign bodies. Non-Secretors do not have this first line of defense; however, their internal defenses are more powerful than Secretors. All of this means that there are some foods that are suitable for Secretors that may not be for Non-Secretors NS and vice versa. To address this, all recipes in this book that are appropriate for Non-Secretors have been tagged as such, and when possible, substitutions are provided to make the other recipes acceptable and healthful for Non-Secretors.

In addition to diet, there are different forms of exercise and stress reduction that are *Beneficial* to each blood type. Those who are Type O require high-intensity exercise for weight loss and stress reduction. So, get moving. Aerobic exercises can be combined with weight training, kickboxing, outdoor sports, hiking, etc. There are plenty of fun ways to work up a sweat and burn off a few calories; just make sure to give it a try three to four times a week for at least thirty to forty minutes each time.

This book is customized for the Type O individual. All recipes are designed to have the most health benefits possible for a Type O, while maintaining flavor and diversity. If you have a SWAMI© Personalized Nutrition Software Program (SWAMI is a proprietary software program designed to produce a unique, one of a kind diet protocol based on your blood type, a series of biometric measurements and your personal history. For more information, see page 250 in the Appendix) and you notice some fruits or vegetables that are an *Avoid* specifically for you, feel free to swap them out for those on your *Beneficial* list. See "Substitutions" for a better idea of what to substitute.

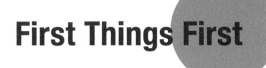

Beneficial Foods

Below is a list of basics to keep in your kitchen; there will be times when meals have to be spontaneous and pretty much thrown together so, if you have essentials from your *Beneficial* and *Neutral* lists on hand, no matter what you make, it will be something that is good for you.

Let's Start with the Fridge

Salad Base

Pick your favorite greens or mix it up each time you go to the grocery store, keeping these salad base options in mind:

BENEFICIALS

Arugula	Boston lettuce	Red leaf lettuce
Bibb lettuce	Escarole	Romaine

These will give you a great start for a last-minute salad, or provide added crunch to a sandwich.

Roasted Vegetables

The best thing you can do for yourself is to keep hearty, fresh vegetables on hand to roast for dinner. Make in bulk to add to the next day's last-minute salad, or add to a frittata for breakfast. Roasted vegetables are a terrific leftover to keep on hand. Most vegetables work well when tossed with olive oil, sea salt, and roasted in a 375-degree oven for 12 to 20 minutes (depending on the size and density of the vegetables.) Here are a few that are both *Beneficial* to Type O and take well to roasting:

 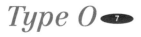

BENEFICIALS

Broccoli	Parsnips	Sweet potatoes
Kale	Peppers	Turnips
Onions	Pumpkin	

Keeping a few of these vegetables in your fridge each week will come in handy and is a perfect way to add more *Beneficials* to your diet.

NEUTRALS

Asparagus	Carrots	Fennel
Beets	Celeriac	Tomatoes
Brussels sprouts	Eggplant	

Fruit

Fruit is a perfect snack paired with nuts or nut butters, but you can also use fruit to make desserts, or add dried fruit to cereal or salads. Some fruits even work well in savory dishes. Below is a list of *Beneficial* fruit for Type O:

BENEFICIALS

Bananas	Figs (dried)	Plums
Blueberries	Guava	Prunes
Cherries	Mango	

Milk

Although Type Os cannot have cow's milk, it's great to have an alternative on hand for smoothies, cereal, some soups, and baked goods. Acceptable milk options for those with Type O:

BENEFICIALS

Almond milk	Rice milk (for Non-Secretor
Hemp milk	Type Os)

Extras

What about those things we all have hanging around in the door of our fridge like salad dressings, condiments, and relishes? Toss all those chemical-heavy bottles and jars and replace them with fresh, tasty, homemade options. Instead of ketchup, which contains vinegar (an *Avoid* for O's), use jarred tomato paste (the jarred kind is a little thinner and doesn't have that

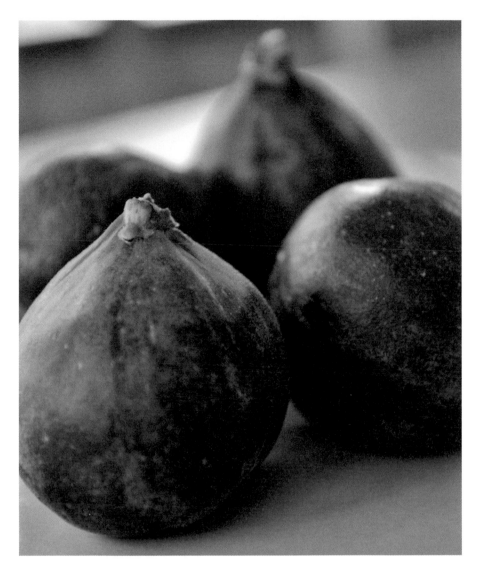

metallic taste from the cans). Tomatoes are highly acidic so they are among the most important foods to avoid buying in cans. The acidity in tomatoes will wear away at the lining of the cans that, in most cases, contains BPA, a hormone-disrupting chemical. Here are a few things that will save your taste buds from boredom:

BENEFICIALS
   Butter or ghee
   Carrot-Ginger Dressing*
   Citrus Dressing*
   Fresh herbs: basil, parsley, oregano, thyme

 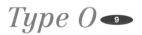

Ground flaxseed
Herb Dressing*
Honey-Mustard Dressing*
Ketchup*
Lemons

*Recipes included in book

Protein

The Type O diet is based on protein consumption, and Type Os are meat eaters who don't need—and don't benefit—from a lot of grains, if any at all. Of course, keeping meat on hand is ideal for your diet. It's a good idea to keep two fresh proteins in the fridge at a time and then two to three in the freezer for backup (more on that later). Below are a few staples that are useful to have on hand.

Please note, all poultry should be organic and all beef should be grass-fed and organic.

BENEFICIALS
Beef tips
Cheeses (feta, goat, mozzarella) If you use SWAMI, there could be cheeses that are more or less *Beneficial* than others, so focus on those.
Eggs
Ground beef (90 percent or leaner)
Lamb steaks (cheaper, and contain more lean meat than chops or rack)
Leftovers (make extra meat and save it for lunch the next day or add to a casserole)
Nut butters (almond, macadamia, pecan, walnut). Almond butter is inexpensive and easily found in supermarkets or natural food stores. Again, if your SWAMI personalized nutrition report indicates one type of nut that is *Beneficial* above the rest, use that one, and make your own nut butter by blending it raw in a high powered food processor until smooth.
Seafood (bass, cod, halibut, perch, pike, rainbow trout, red snapper, sole, sturgeon, swordfish, tilefish, yellowtail)
Turkey tenderloins
Chicken

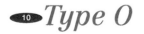

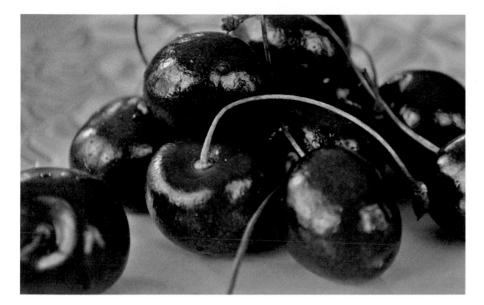

Filling up Your Freezer

Smoothies

A smoothie is a great alternative for breakfast or a perfect, protein-filled snack. Smoothies are great go-to recipes, so make sure to have ingredients for them at all times. Of course, use seasonal, fresh fruit as well. For a thicker consistency, mix in some frozen fruits and vegetables. Here are a few *Beneficial* options:

BENEFICIALS

Blueberries	Kale	Spinach
Cherries	Mango	

NEUTRALS

Peaches	Strawberries (Avoid for Type O
Pineapple	Non-Secretors)
Raspberries	

Leftovers

It is always helpful to double the recipe when making foods that freeze easily such as:

Chili	Cookies

Crackers	Pesto
Lasagna	Sauces
Muffins	Stews
Pasta sauce	

Pesto can be stored in BPA-free ice cube trays for individual servings. In the following pages you will find more information on safe food storage as well as suggestions for cooking in bulk.

Proteins

Just like keeping fresh protein sources in your fridge, it is always helpful to keep at least a few options in the freezer as well. To defrost meats/poultry or seafood, take them out the day before and put them in the refrigerator. Listed below are terrific options to store in the freezer:

BENEFICIALS
Beef tips
Ground beef (90 percent or leaner)
Lamb steaks (cheaper, and contain more lean meat than chops or rack)
Seafood (bass, cod, halibut, perch, pike, red snapper, rainbow
    trout, sole, sturgeon, swordfish, tilefish, yellowtail)
Turkey tenderloins/Ground turkey
Chicken

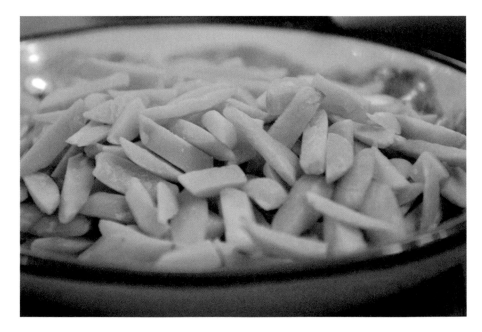

Time to Get in That Pantry

Snacks

The first thing we all go into the pantry for is a quick bite on the run or to pack a snack to ship off to school with the kids. It is important that these midday treats are balanced and wholesome. The best way to make sure that happens is to stock your pantry well.

Here are a few staples for Type O:

Almond butter
Brown rice cakes
Dark chocolate (70 percent or higher)
Dried fruit (cranberries, cherries, figs, prunes)
Fresh fruit (bananas, cherries, plums, mangoes)
Nuts (almonds, macadamia, pecans, walnuts)
Pumpkin seeds

If you want to prep ahead for those times when you are in a rush, make individual servings of combinations of nuts, dried fruit, and maybe even a little dark chocolate. Store in small, resealable glass containers and take them in the car, on the plane, or anywhere you are headed.

Drinks

Drinking water is always the best option, but when you want to add a little flavor to your beverage repertoire, dabble in these *Beneficial* teas and try them plain, with some seltzer, or with a touch of lemon/lime or mint. (There are also a few recipes for teas and seltzer in this book.)

BENEFICIALS

Chamomile tea
Dandelion tea
Ginger tea
Green tea

Licorice tea
Mint tea
Seltzer

Grains/Legumes

As mentioned earlier, grains are not really meant for those following the Type O diet. In moderation, however, the grains listed below are terrific.

Quinoa, for example, cooks in 12 minutes and is a light but filling side for a fast, weeknight dinner. Beans are a perfect addition to add satiating proteins and carbohydrates to salads, casseroles, stews, dips, and soups.

BENEFICIALS

Adzuki beans	Millet
Black-eyed peas	Quinoa
Brown rice	Red Quinoa

Seasonings

Making healthy food taste good is non-negotiable. One quick trick to doing so is to know the way around your spice cabinet. Herbs and spices are calorie-free and flavor packed. The spices listed below also happen to be terrific for your Type O body. Keep a jar of Basic Gluten-Free Bread Crumbs NS on hand for a quick topping on a casserole, to bread seafood or poultry, and to add to meat loaf. Additionally, as much as you would like to repress your sweet tooth, it is an unrealistic expectation for most, so stock up on natural sweeteners like agave and maple syrup, but use sparingly.

BENEFICIALS

Agave nectar

Basic Gluten-Free Bread Crumbs NS

Maple syrup

Olive oil

Spices (allspice, basil, cardamom, cayenne, chili powder, cinnamon, cumin, curry, garlic, oregano, paprika, parsley, sage, salt, tarragon, thyme, turmeric)

Recipe Ideas for Last-Minute Cooking

Time-Saving Tricks

Make these recipes in bulk and store in your freezer to grab on the go: flax chips, smoothies in individual portions, baked goods, chili, granola, soups, casseroles, pasta sauce, pesto (in ice-cube trays), and stews.

When making dressings or condiments, double or triple the recipe and store the extra in the refrigerator. If you are making the recipe with one lemon, you might as well do it with three and save yourself the prep and cleanup again and again.

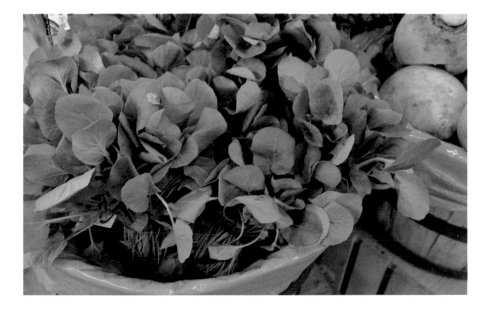

Utilize Roasted Vegetables

Let's reemphasize here how useful leftover roasted vegetables can be. Not only are they ready to be thrown into just about any dish, but they also add tremendous flavor with little effort. Here are a few examples where you can toss in roasted vegetables and have a tasty new dish:

Casseroles	Omelets	Soufflés
Cold pasta salads	Pizzas	Spring rolls
Crêpes	Quiches	Tacos
Frittatas	Rice salads	Vegetable tarts
Lettuce wraps	Salads	

Next time you make roasted vegetables for dinner, do yourself a favor and double up on that recipe.

Review Your Stock

Now that you have the basics, it's time to take a look at some of the *Avoids*. You have lived your whole life eating whatever you want. Now you open your cabinets and think, how do I start over? The answer is simple: you don't have to. You just have to emphasize the healthy choices that you are now privy to. But you should ditch anything that is categorized *Best Avoided* for your type. Listed below are a few places where *Avoids* may be lurking and ready to sabotage your otherwise perfect, new diet.

- Open up the fridge—take inventory of all condiments, sauces, stocks, and other processed foods.
- Open the pantry—familiarize yourself with ingredients in your snacks, cereals, pastas, spices, and other foods.
- Open the freezer—remove frozen dinners. Just do it. You can be sure they are not doing you any good. Other than that, the same applies here as above—evaluate what you have, and review ingredients just to get yourself acquainted with what you are dealing with.

Once you have done that, take out all questionable foods and line them up on the counter or table. Refer to the Type O diet in *Eat Right 4 Your Type*, *Live Right 4 Your Type*, the *Blood Type O Food, Beverage and Supplements Lists* book, or you can use Type Base Food Values online (www.dadamo.com). If you have taken the next step and used the SWAMI Personalized Nutrition Software program, refer to your SWAMI food lists in your reference book. Check out your *Avoids*, as this will be the most efficient way of eliminating those foods.

Now that you are familiar with what you must *Avoid* and have removed possible violators from your pantry, fridge, and freezer, let's go through some of the main offenders one at a time.

Please note that *Avoids* are not limited to the examples listed below.

Vinegar

Type Os are not vinegar friendly. The thought of living without vinegar can sound impossible at first, but the many recipes in this book will fill that gap in your diet. Be sure to get it out of your kitchen—out of sight, out of mind. So, the big question is, where does vinegar lurk when the word *vinegar* is not in the name—as in balsamic, red wine, apple cider, or rice wine vinegars?

The following foods contain vinegar:

All vinegars (red, white, apple cider, balsamic, rice, etc.)	Mayonnaise
	Olives
Chili sauces	Pickled vegetables
Cocktails sauce	Pickles
Ketchup	Prepared horseradish

Prepared mustard   Steak sauce
Relishes   Soy sauce
Salad dressings   Worcestershire sauce

Wheat/Gluten

It may feel traumatizing but it's better to face the facts: wheat is not good for you—and for many Type Os, neither is gluten. Wheat is used in a surprising number of places, however, so let's figure out how to eliminate it first and then tackle the strategies to throw it away and never look back.

Many wheat-free grains are also gluten-free. Gluten is the protein found in wheat, rye, and barley. It is a tricky ingredient to replace because it plays a large role in what makes bread so irresistible. It creates elasticity in dough that holds bread together, and provides height and that "pull it apart" chewy texture. Grains that lack this protein, such as rice, buckwheat, quinoa, amaranth, and teff have a tendency to taste grainy, fall apart while cooking, and do not rise easily. Do not let this discourage you; You should know the facts in case you decide to make something using your newly allowable grains and the recipe does not initially turn out the way you'd hoped. There are recipes included in this book for scones, breads, muffins, pancakes, and even waffles that will have you satisfied and maybe even ready to do your own experimenting. Working with these grains can be exciting because they bring different flavors to the table that you cannot get from wheat, so dive in and enjoy.

A few places wheat (and gluten) exist:

Baking powder (some)   Cookies
Beer   Corn bread
Blue cheese (some)   Couscous
Bread crumbs   Crackers
Breaded fish   Croutons
Breads   Dumplings
Brewer's yeast   Farina
Broth (some)   Flavored extract (some)
Bulgur   Food starch or modified food
Candies (some)   starch (some)
Caramel color (some)   Graham flour
Cereal   Gravy
Chewing gum   Hot dogs
Cold cuts (some)   Hushpuppies

Hydrolyzed plant protein
Hydrolyzed vegetable protein
Ice cream (some)
Kamut
Malt (flavoring, and vinegar)
Matzo
Meat loaf
Meatballs
"Natural flavor" (either soy or gluten)
Pancakes/waffles
Pasta
Pastries
Pie crust
Pitas
Pizza crust
Potato chips (some)
Pretzels
Salad dressings
Seitan
Semolina
Soups
Soy sauce
Spice mixtures (some)
Syrup
Tamari
Teriyaki sauce
Textured vegetable protein
Wheat
Wheat protein
Worcestershire sauce

A list of foods and ingredients that will help to replace much of the list above is provided in the substitutions section.

Corn

Corn is the source of arguably the greatest food debate of the century. The movie *Food Inc.* came out and exposed many people to how the mass production of corn has become a national, if not global, issue. With the introduction of genetically modified organisms (GMOs) or foods that are genetically altered to optimize their growing potential, corn, quite literally, became another species. As an *Avoid* for Type O, eliminating corn provides yet another opportunity to clean up your diet. It is used in a wide range of processed goods in this country, making it difficult to avoid altogether. We've tried to highlight where corn is generally hidden, but know that with this diet, it is okay to run into an *Avoid* once in a while without sabotaging your progress. If you are not acutely sick and are simply using the Blood Type Diet for general health, you only have to be 80 percent compliant to see 100 percent results. How forgiving is that?

The following are a few places corn exists:

Alcohol (some)
Artificial flavorings
Artificial sweeteners
Ascorbic acid
Aspartame
Baked goods

Baking powder (some)	Malt/malt syrup
Canned fruits	Modified food starch
Canned vegetables	Molasses (some)
Caramel color	Polenta
Cereal	Popcorn
Cheese spreads	Prepared mustard (some)
Citric acid	Salad dressings
Confectioners' sugar	Salt (iodized)
Corn flour	Soda
Corn syrup	Splenda
Cornstarch	Sucrose
Fast food	Sugar (if not cane or beet)
Food starch	Sweet beverages (containing
Grits	corn syrup)
Hominy	Tacos
Hydrolyzed vegetable protein	Tomato sauce (with corn syrup)
Ice cream (some)	Vitamins (some)
Instant coffee/tea	Xanthan gum
Ketchup	Yeast (some)
Licorice	Yogurt (with corn syrup)
Maize	

The Rest

Other than vinegar, wheat, gluten, and corn, determining what to take out of your cabinets/fridge/freezer will be straightforward. Take the time to go through your list of *Avoids* and remove them from your house. If you have canned goods and non-perishables, you can donate to your local food bank. To find a food bank in your area, go to: http://feedingamerica.org. But, again, unless you are acutely sick and can apply the 80/20 rule to save money, you can phase out the *Avoids* by only eating them once in a while until they are gone and then filling your cabinets with only *Neutrals* and *Beneficials*.

Now you are ready to go to the store and grab a few essentials to fill in the gaps.

How to Read These Recipes

This cookbook is designed to be as practical and helpful to the Blood Type dieter as possible. We took into consideration that many families could be

 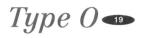

cooking for multiple blood types or preparing meals for friends with varying blood types. In order to make doing so practical, each of the *Eat Right 4 Your Type* cookbooks contains the same or similar recipe ideas with different executions to suit the needs of each blood type. Though the recipe titles in each book are nearly identical, ingredients and methods might vary quite a bit. There are many recipes that are *Beneficial* across the board and are marked with an (A/B/AB/O) to identify that they are universal to every type. For example, every blood type has a pancake recipe; however, the recipe for Type Os has grains to *Avoid* that might be on the *Beneficial* list for other types, so each recipe contains different flours. Every recipe is also written to contain as many *Beneficial* foods as possible while maintaining that taste is still of the utmost importance. After all, you are not going to be inclined to dive into a kale cookie or a seaweed hot cocoa, but you won't be able to resist the spicy seafood stew with wakame, which tastes like it is fresh from the sea. The point is, we want you coming back for more each time so you see that eating for your blood type is as far from sacrifice as indulging in a bar of chocolate.

As you make your way through this book, you will notice that once in a while there is a highlighted section called "Featured Ingredient." There are several ingredients used in this book that you may not have come across before, some that are *Beneficial* for your diet and some that are beneficial for your taste buds. In an effort to familiarize you with these ingredients, there is a brief summary explaining a little about what that ingredient is and how or why it is used. Don't be afraid to experiment with unfamiliar territory.

Many people who follow the Blood Type Diet have come to my office or used the tests on my website (www. dadamo.com) to create an individual diet plan. If you have done that, you have a SWAMI Personalized Nutrition book that may vary slightly from the general Type O diet because it takes into consideration family and medical history, Secretor Status, and Geno-Type. (The GenoType is a further refinement of my work in personalized nutrition. It uses a variety of simple measurements, combined with blood type status to classify individuals as one of six basic Epigenotypes: The Hunter, Gatherer, Teacher, Explorer, Warrior, and Nomad types.) Due to the variations in *Beneficial*, *Neutral*, and *Best Avoided* foods, there may be some recipes containing ingredients that do not suit you as an individual. Please do not skip these recipes entirely. There is always a way to make quick and easy substitutions. (See "Substitutions," page 227.) As a quick piece of advice, however, vegetables can be easily swapped out—leafy greens for other leafy greens, specific type of beans for another. In some cases, an ingredient can be simply omitted from the recipe if the *Avoid* is not a star component. Additionally, if a recipe appears too spicy for your taste, simply reduce the amount of spice used. The same principle applies if you just can't get enough spice; simply amp it up where you see fit.

You will see that recipes are also tagged according to Secretor Status. Some recipes are not appropriate for Non-Secretors but are fine for Secretors (see legend on the following page). In most instances when this is the case, there are simple substitutions to adapt the recipe for Non-Secretors. In a few cases, however, the recipe will be an *Avoid* altogether for a Type O Non-Secretor. For example, cheese is tricky for Non-Secretors. There are no cheeses that are universally appropriate for all Type O Non-Secretors, but manchego is *Neutral* for some. Therefore, you'll see manchego often used as a substitute for Non-Secretors. If you try manchego and it does not work for you, simply omit all cheese from the recipe.

In many of the recipes in this book, you will see sea salt written as "sea salt, to taste" and might be wondering what that means or how much to add. Salt can make or break your dish; if you add too much, there is no going back. Try adding a little at a time, taste, and add more if needed. What is *a little*? Start with pinching a bit between your fingers and sprinkling it into your dish, give it a minute to incorporate, and then taste. If you were to measure a pinch, it would be a little less than ⅛ of a teaspoon.

As you know at this point, one of the major changes for people following the Type O diet is becoming wheat- (and for some) gluten-free. Throughout the book, recipes containing flour often use multiple types of flour for each recipe. Why not simply swap wheat flour for rice flour? The problem with wheat-/gluten-free baking is that the result can yield a grainy and dense product that does not hold together well. As a way to combat these issues, you can combine different wheat-/gluten-free flours that have various textures and tastes, and react differently to moisture. The idea of eating one type of anything repeatedly for life sounds like a bad idea. Each type of grain provides a different set of nutrients, fiber, and sugars, which in turn enrich your body in different ways. In order to reduce the hassle of using multiple grains in baking, the best advice is to buy glass or ceramic canisters to store a few of your most frequently used flours (such as brown rice, tapioca or arrowroot starch, teff, or millet) and keep them in an accessible place, like your countertop. That way when you want to make pancakes, you can quickly scoop ⅓ cup from each canister, mix together, and be ready to cook.

Remember to read each recipe in its entirety before starting to ensure you know how much time it will take and if there are any ingredients you

 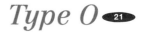

will need to buy ahead of time. Finally, enjoy making, eating, and sharing these recipes.

RECIPE LEGEND:

- An * is used when a recipe ingredient needs further instruction, substitution, or comment. This information is found at the bottom of a recipe.
- All recipes are appropriate for Type O Secretors.
- **NS** represents a recipe that is appropriate for Type O Non-Secretors.
- Recipe ingredients that are NOT appropriate for Type O Non-Secretors **NS** are notated with appropriate acceptable substitutions within recipe ingredients.
- **S** (S Only!) represents a recipe that is appropriate for Type O Secretors only.

A REVIEW OF THE FOOD LISTS:

Throughout this book we refer to a number of places to find the comprehensive foods lists for the Blood Type Diet. Here's a recap of where you can find the lists so you can use the one that is right for you:

- *Eat Right 4 Your Type*, which provides the entry point into the Blood Type Diet
- *Live Right 4 Your Type*, which incorporates the value of the Secretor Status
- *Blood Type O Food, Beverage, and Supplement Lists* from *Eat Right 4 Your Type*, a handy pocket guide with the basic food lists
- *Change Your Genetic Destiny* (originally published as *The Geno-Type Diet*, which provides a further refinement of the diet by using blood type, secretor status, and a series of biometric measurements to further individualize your food lists
- SWAMI Personalized Nutrition Software, designed to harness the power of computers and artificial intelligence, using their tremendous precision and speed to help tailor unique, one-of-a-kind diets. From its extensive knowledge base, SWAMI can evaluate over 700 foods for over 200 individual attributes (such as cholesterol level, gluten content, presence of antioxidants, etc.) to determine if that food is either a superfood or toxin for you. It provides a specific, unique diet in an easy-to-read, user friendly format, complete with food lists, recipes, and meal planning.

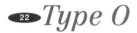

Breakfast

Quinoa Muesli ■ *Blackstrap-Cherry Granola* NS ■ *Granola–Nut Butter Fruit Slices* ■ *Breakfast Egg Salad* ■ *Turkey Bacon–Spinach Squares* ■ *Swiss Chard and Cremini Frittata* NS ■ *Broccoli-Feta Frittata* ■ *Maple-Sausage Scramble* ■ *Homemade Turkey Breakfast Sausage* ■ *Savory Herb and Cheese Bread Pudding* ■ *Spinach-Zucchini Soufflé* ■ *Cinnamon-Millet Crêpes* ■ *Brown Rice Pancakes* ■ *Wild-Rice Waffles* ■ *Pumpkin Muffins with Carob Drizzle* ■ *Pear-Rosemary Bread* NS ■ *Cherry Scones* ■ *Blueberry-Macadamia Muffins*

Breakfast recipes were written with diversity in mind so that you do not end up eating the same thing every day. The idea here is to alternate: eggs one day, quinoa or granola the next, and so on in order to keep providing your body with different nutrients each day. You will probably notice the biggest change in these recipes is the types of flour used. Don't be intimidated; try one simple recipe like Brown Rice Pancakes to get your feet wet and move on to the rest. Once you have the new flour on hand, the rest is just like any other recipe.

Quinoa Muesli

½ cup quinoa

½ cup water

½ cup almond milk plus more if needed (NS substitute rice milk)

¼ teaspoon sea salt

2 tablespoons dried cherries

1 tablespoon dried cranberries

2 tablespoons slivered almonds

2 tablespoons chopped walnuts

¼ teaspoon cinnamon (NS omit cinnamon)

2 teaspoons maple syrup (NS substitute 1 teaspoon of molasses and 1 teaspoon agave)

¼ cup crunchy rice cereal

1. Rinse quinoa. Combine quinoa, water, almond milk, sea salt, cherries, and cranberries in a small saucepan, and bring to a boil. Cook 10 minutes, remove from heat, and let sit an additional 4 to 5 minutes. Quinoa will absorb all the water and become light and fluffy when done.

2. While the quinoa cooks, toast almonds and walnuts in a dry skillet over medium heat for 2 minutes or until slightly golden brown. Watch nuts carefully, as they have a tendency to burn easily because of their high fat content.

3. Fluff cooked quinoa with a fork and add toasted nuts, cinnamon, if using, and maple syrup. Top with crunchy rice cereal, and add more almond milk, if desired.

4. Serve immediately.

▶ SERVES 2

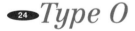

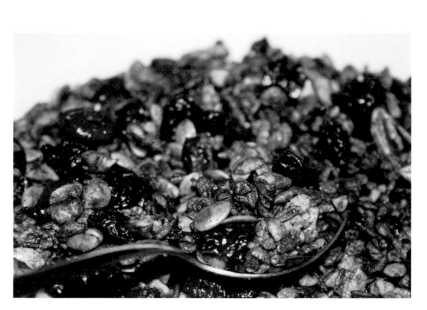

Blackstrap-Cherry Granola NS

4 cups crispy rice cereal

1 cup chopped walnuts

1 cup chopped pecans

¼ cup whole flaxseed

¼ cup blackstrap molasses

2 teaspoons olive oil

1 tablespoon agave

⅛ teaspoon sea salt

¼ cup water

1 cup halved dried cherries

½ cup halved dried cranberries

1. Preheat oven to 350 degrees. Line a baking sheet with parchment paper and set aside.

2. In a large bowl, combine rice cereal, walnuts, pecans, and flaxseed, and set aside.

3. In a small saucepan, combine molasses, olive oil, agave, salt, and water. Heat over medium heat for 2 minutes, whisking to combine.

4. Pour molasses mixture over granola mixture, toss to coat, and spread onto prepared sheet pan. Bake 10 minutes.

5. Reduce oven temperature to 300 degrees. Stir granola, and place back in the oven. Bake an additional 25 minutes.

6. Toss granola with cherries and cranberries.

7. Serve warm, or cool fully and store in an airtight, glass container for up to 2 weeks or in the freezer for up to 2 months.

▶ MAKES 32 (¼-CUP) SERVINGS

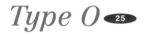

Granola–Nut Butter Fruit Slices

3 tablespoons almond butter

⅓ cup granola*

¼ teaspoon ground cinnamon (NS omit cinnamon)

Sea salt, to taste

1 pear

1 apple (NS substitute banana)

1 lemon

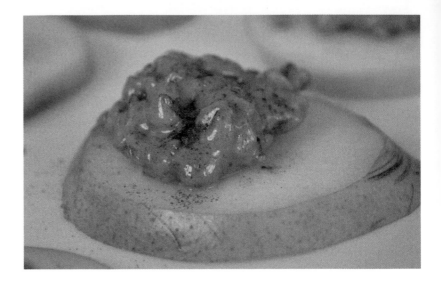

1. Stir almond butter, granola, cinnamon, if using, and salt until granola is evenly coated, and set aside.

2. Thinly slice fruit into ¼-inch rounds. Cut lemon in half, and rub cut side on fruit pieces to prevent browning. (NS slice banana in half lengthwise and then across.)

3. Spoon 1 to 2 teaspoons of the granola mixture on each fruit slice and enjoy.

*See Blackstrap-Cherry Granola NS recipe (page 25).

▶ SERVES 4

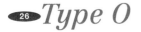

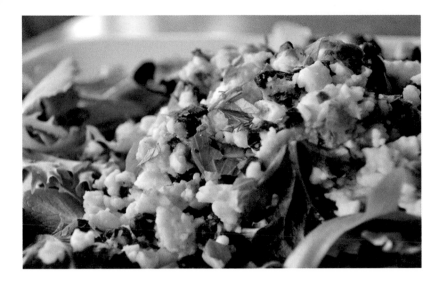

Breakfast Egg Salad

1. In a separate bowl, whisk together dressing ingredients, and set aside.

2. Heat olive oil in a small skillet over medium heat. Toast black-eyed peas for 2 to 3 minutes, until warm and slightly crunchy.

3. Remove eggs from shells, and use a fork to break apart in a bowl. Add beans, cheese, and parsley to eggs, and toss with dressing. Serve over mixed baby greens.

▶ SERVES 4

dressing:

½ teaspoon mustard powder

1 tablespoon olive oil

1 tablespoon lemon juice

1 tablespoon onion, grated

Sea salt, to taste

2 teaspoons olive oil

½ cup cooked or canned black-eyed peas, drained and rinsed

3 large hard-boiled eggs

¼ cup grated mozzarella cheese (NS omit cheese)

1 tablespoon chopped parsley

2 cups mixed baby greens

Sea salt, to taste

Type O 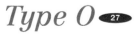 27

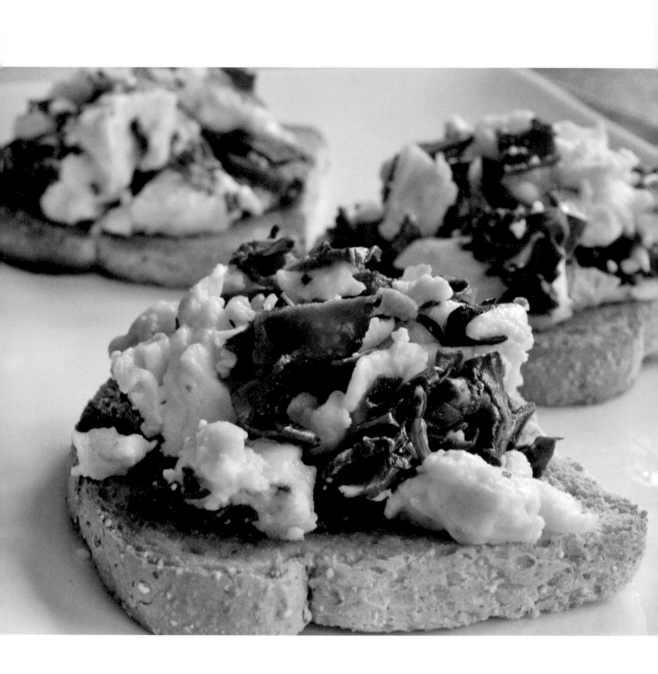

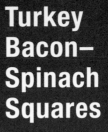
1. Heat a large skillet over medium heat and spray with nonstick cooking spray.

2. Once the skillet is hot, add bacon and cook 3 to 4 minutes. Flip and cook an additional 2 to 3 minutes, until bacon is crispy. Remove from pan and let cool, then crumble and set aside.

3. Whisk eggs and egg whites in a small bowl, and set aside. In the same skillet used for bacon, add olive oil and reduce heat slightly. Add spinach and sauté 2 minutes. Add sea salt, to taste. Pour eggs over spinach, cooking gently and stirring until done, about 2 additional minutes. Turn off heat and add reserved bacon and cheese.

4. Spoon mixture on toast, and serve immediately.

▶ **SERVES 4**

3 strips turkey bacon

3 large eggs

3 large egg whites

2 teaspoons olive oil

2 cups fresh spinach

Sea salt, to taste

¼ cup mozzarella cheese (**NS** omit cheese)

4 slices brown rice/millet bread, toasted

tip: If the bacon is not as crispy as you like, drizzle a touch of olive oil into the pan while cooking, to help it along.

featured ingredient

turkey bacon (nitrate- /preservative-free)

Not all turkey bacon is the same. There are many types/brands on the market, but most are artificially derived, loaded with salt and preservatives, and full of nitrates . . . all things you absolutely do not want to be eating. There are a few companies that make turkey bacon without these unhealthy and artificial additives, which can be found at your local natural foods store and in some mainstream grocery stores.

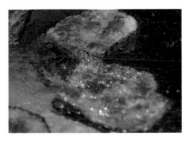

Swiss Chard and Cremini Frittata (NS)

2 teaspoons ghee

¼ cup finely diced Spanish onion

1 cup diced cremini mushrooms

3 cups chopped Swiss chard

3 large eggs

3 large egg whites

2 tablespoons brown rice flour

Sea salt, to taste

1 teaspoon chopped fresh tarragon

1 teaspoon olive oil

1 tablespoon pepitas (pumpkin seeds), toasted

1. Preheat oven to 375 degrees.

2. Heat ghee in a heatproof sauté pan over medium heat. Sauté onion, mushrooms, and Swiss chard for 4 to 5 minutes, until vegetables become tender.

3. In a large bowl, whisk together eggs, egg whites, brown rice flour, salt, and tarragon. Add olive oil to skillet, pour egg mixture over vegetables, and cook for 1 minute.

4. Transfer to the oven, and bake 6 to 8 minutes, or until firm and edges are golden. Top with pepitas, and serve warm.

▶ SERVES 4

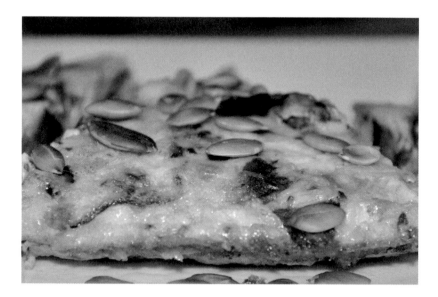

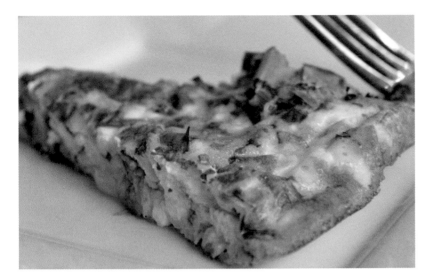

Broccoli-Feta Frittata

1 head broccoli

¼ teaspoon sea salt, divided

1 tablespoon plus 2 teaspoons olive oil

3 large eggs

2 large egg whites

⅓ cup crumbled feta (NS omit cheese)

½ cup chopped spinach

¼ cup finely diced chives

2 teaspoons brown rice flour

1 tablespoon chopped oregano

1. Preheat oven to 375 degrees.

2. Dice broccoli into bite-size pieces and place in a single layer on a baking sheet. Sprinkle with a dash of sea salt and 1 tablespoon olive oil. Bake 15 minutes, remove from oven, and set aside. Turn oven temperature to Broil setting.

3. In a medium-size bowl, whisk eggs, egg whites, feta, spinach, chives, flour, oregano, and remaining salt until well combined.

4. Brush remaining 2 teaspoons olive oil across a heatproof medium-size skillet over medium heat, to create a nonstick surface. Once warm, add egg mixture to hot pan with broccoli. Cook 1 to 2 minutes, lifting the side of the eggs gently with your spatula to encourage uncooked egg to run down into the bottom of the skillet.

5. If the handle of your skillet is rubber, wrap tightly with tinfoil to prevent melting. Place skillet under broiler for 2 minutes, or until the eggs set and brown very slightly on the edges.

6. Serve warm.

▶ SERVES 4

 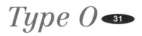

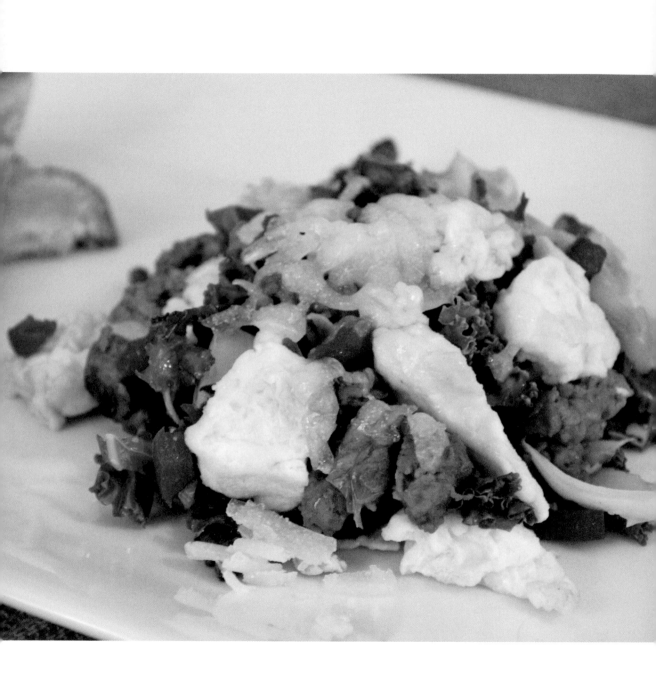

Maple-Sausage Scramble

1. Heat 2 teaspoons olive oil in a large skillet over medium heat. Sauté onion, kale, artichokes, and peppers over medium heat, 5-6 minutes. Remove vegetables from skillet and set aside. Add remaining 1 teaspoon olive oil to skillet and brown turkey sausage, breaking into bite-size pieces until cooked through, 5 to 6 minutes. Drizzle with maple syrup and stir to combine. Add to vegetables and set aside.

2. Whisk eggs and egg whites with water and salt then add to skillet, reducing the heat to medium-low. Stir gently with a heat-safe spatula until firm and cooked through. Add sausage mixture back to skillet and stir to combine.

3. Serve topped with shredded cheese.

▶ **SERVES 4**

1 tablespoon olive oil, divided

¼ cup finely chopped white onion

3 cups chopped kale

2 cups frozen, quartered artichoke hearts, thawed

⅓ cup finely diced red bell pepper

½ pound raw turkey sausage

1 tablespoon maple syrup (NS substitute 1 teaspoon agave and 1 teaspoon molasses)

3 large eggs

2 large egg whites

1 tablespoon water

Sea salt, to taste

¼ cup shredded mozzarella cheese (NS substitute manchego cheese or omit cheese)

Homemade Turkey Breakfast Sausage

2 teaspoons olive oil

½ cup finely diced onion

½ cup finely diced fennel

1 pound ground turkey

1 teaspoon fennel seed

1 teaspoon paprika

1 teaspoon sea salt

¼ teaspoon chili powder

1 clove garlic, minced

½ cup finely diced Bosc pear

2 teaspoons maple syrup (NS substitute agave)

1. In a large sauté pan, heat olive oil over medium heat. Add onion and fennel and sauté 4 to 5 minutes, or until tender. Remove from heat and let cool to room temperature, about 10 minutes.

2. Combine turkey with fennel seed, paprika, salt, chili powder, garlic, pear, maple syrup, and cooled vegetables in a large bowl. Use your hands to incorporate all ingredients into the meat, being careful not to over mix.

3. Form meat into small, hot dog–shaped links. Spray a medium skillet with olive oil non-stick cooking spray. Cook links 8 to 10 minutes over medium heat or until meat is browned on all sides, inside of the sausage is no longer pink, and juices run clear.

4. Serve warm alone or alongside scrambled eggs for a protein-packed breakfast.

▶ SERVES 4

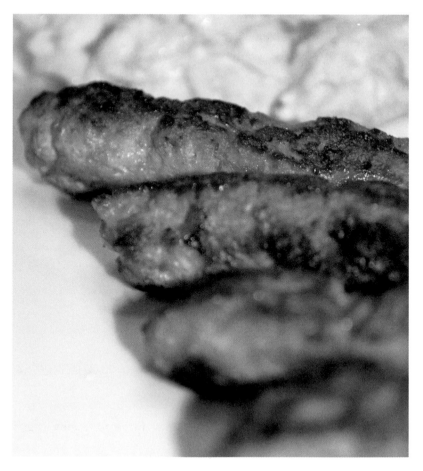

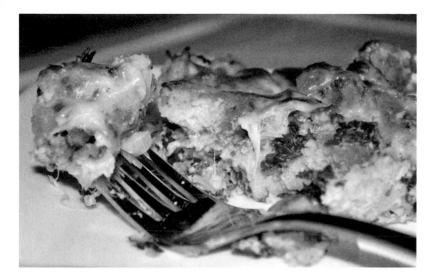

Savory Herb and Cheese Bread Pudding

1. Preheat oven to 350 degrees. Spray a 9" x 11" baking dish with nonstick cooking spray and set aside.

2. Heat olive oil and ghee in a large skillet over medium heat. Sauté onion, mushrooms, zucchini, and kale just until tender, about 5 to 6 minutes. Season with salt, to taste, and set aside.

3. Spread bread cubes on a baking sheet in a single layer. Toast for 3 to 4 minutes until slightly golden brown. Toss in a large bowl with vegetables.

4. Whisk together almond milk, stock, eggs, thyme, rosemary, and sage. Pour over bread and vegetables and toss. Pour the entire mixture into prepared baking dish. Top with mozzarella cheese and bake, covered, for 35 minutes.

5. Uncover and bake an additional 10 minutes, until cheese is bubbling and slightly brown.

6. Serve warm.

*See Vegetable Stock **NS** recipe (page 223).

▶ SERVES 12

2 teaspoons olive oil

1 teaspoon ghee

2 cups diced onion

2 cups quartered cremini mushrooms

2 cups diced zucchini

6 cups torn kale

Sea salt, to taste

8 cups brown rice/millet bread cubes (about 8–10 slices)

1 cup almond milk (**NS** substitute rice milk)

1 cup Vegetable Stock*

4 large eggs, beaten

1 teaspoon fresh thyme

1 teaspoon fresh rosemary, chopped

1 teaspoon fresh sage, chopped

1 cup mozzarella cheese (**NS** substitute manchego cheese or omit)

tip: Cremini mushrooms are also known as baby portabella mushrooms.

Spinach-Zucchini Soufflé

1 tablespoon ghee

2 tablespoons brown rice flour

½ cup almond milk (NS substitute rice milk)

½ cup Vegetable Stock*

2 cups packed spinach

2 cups chopped zucchini

2 large egg yolks

¼ cup chopped basil

¼ cup crumbled feta cheese (NS omit cheese)

⅛ teaspoon ground cloves

4 large egg whites, room temperature

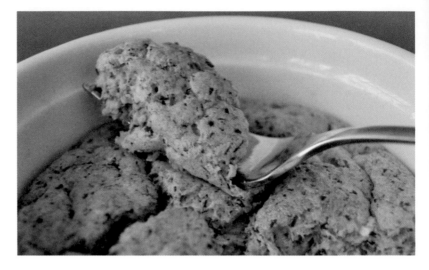

1. Preheat oven to 350 degrees. Spray 4 (12-oz.) ramekins with nonstick cooking spray and set aside.

2. Melt ghee in a saucepan over medium heat, and whisk in flour. Gradually add milk and stock, whisking continuously until thickened, about 3 to 4 minutes. Once mixture is thick and resembles the consistency of yogurt, remove from heat and cool completely.

3. Shred spinach and zucchini in a food processor, and strain excess liquid through cheesecloth or a paper towel. Place vegetables in a bowl, and whisk in egg yolks, basil, cheese, and cloves. Fold milk mixture into vegetable mixture, and set aside.

4. In a dry, glass bowl, beat egg whites with a hand mixer until they form stiff peaks. Fold the egg whites, one-third at a time, into the vegetables. Divide mixture evenly among prepared ramekins. Set ramekins on a baking dish, and fill the baking dish halfway with hot water. Carefully place in the oven and bake for 45 minutes or until tester comes out clean.

5. Serve immediately.

*See Vegetable Stock NS recipe (page 223).

▶ SERVES 4

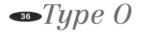
EAT RIGHT FOR YOUR TYPE PERSONALIZED COOKBOOK

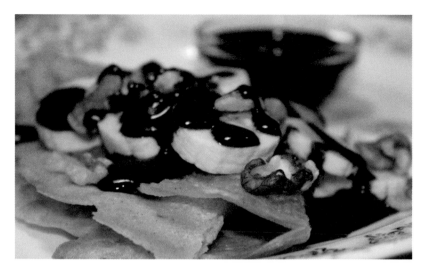

Cinnamon-Millet Crêpes

¾ cup millet flour

¼ cup brown rice flour

½ teaspoon sea salt

¼ teaspoon cinnamon (NS omit cinnamon)

1¼ cups almond milk (NS substitute rice milk)

1 large egg

1 tablespoon plus 1 teaspoon ghee, melted and cooled, divided

1. In a medium bowl, whisk together flours, sea salt, and cinnamon.

2. In a separate bowl, beat almond milk, egg, and 1 tablespoon ghee. Add to flour mixture, and whisk until well blended. Cover and let sit 1 hour in the refrigerator.

3. Heat a large sauté pan over medium heat, and brush remaining 1 teaspoon ghee evenly across the bottom of the pan. Using a ¼-cup measure, scoop batter into pan and quickly turn in circular motions to spread the batter into a very thin layer. Let cook 1 minute or until the batter firms and edges lift slightly off the pan. Use an offset spatula to flip, and cook 1 additional minute. Repeat with remaining batter.

4. Serve with Chocolate Syrup NS (page 219), walnuts, and fresh-sliced banana.

▶ SERVES 4

tip: When adding ghee or butter to eggs, let it cool to room temperature after melting so that the heat does not scramble the eggs.

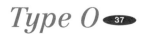

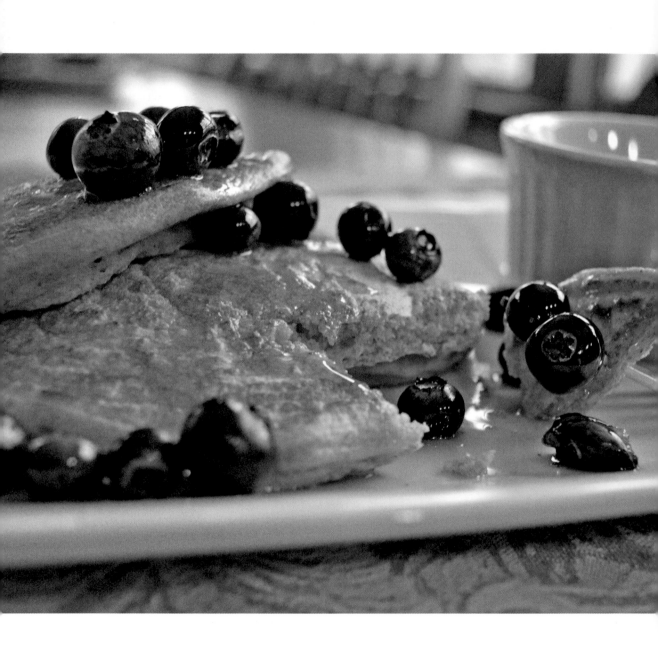

1. Preheat oven to 200 degrees.

2. In a bowl, whisk flours, baking powder, and salt until combined. Set aside.

3. Mash banana with ghee in a separate bowl. Whisk in egg, egg white, and milk.

4. Add wet ingredients to dry ingredients and mix until combined and free of lumps.

5. Heat a skillet over medium heat and coat with nonstick spray. Using a ¼-cup measure, spoon batter into pan and cook 1 to 2 minutes, until small bubbles appear on surface and the edges begin to lift slightly off the bottom of the pan. Flip pancakes and cook 1 additional minute. Repeat with remaining batter.

6. Keep pancakes warm in the oven, draped with a slightly damp paper towel or clean kitchen towel. Serve warm.

▶ SERVES 4

tip: Refillable spray cans are widely available, so fill with allowable oil and use as nonstick spray. Use light olive oil as a go-to oil in your refillable spray can. Olive oil is a *Beneficial* food, and if you use light instead of extra virgin, it won't impart much taste—something you want out of a nonstick spray.

Brown Rice Pancakes

⅔ cup brown rice flour

⅓ cup tapioca flour (NS substitute arrowroot starch or white rice flour)

2 teaspoons baking powder

½ teaspoon sea salt

⅓ banana, mashed

1 tablespoon ghee or butter

1 large egg

1 large egg white

⅔ cup almond milk (NS substitute rice milk)

featured ingredient

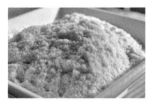

brown rice flour

Brown rice flour is made by milling brown rice into a fine flour. Hearty with a mild flavor, brown rice flour is used in this book as a base for most gluten-free baking. When left to its own devices, however, brown rice flour has a tendency to taste grainy and cause baked goods to deflate after baking. Pairing brown rice flour with a very fine, almost powder-like grain such as tapioca or arrowroot starch will contribute greatly to evening out the final product's texture. Brown rice is a *Neutral* food for Type O, and should be eaten in moderation for weight-loss purposes.

 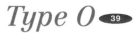

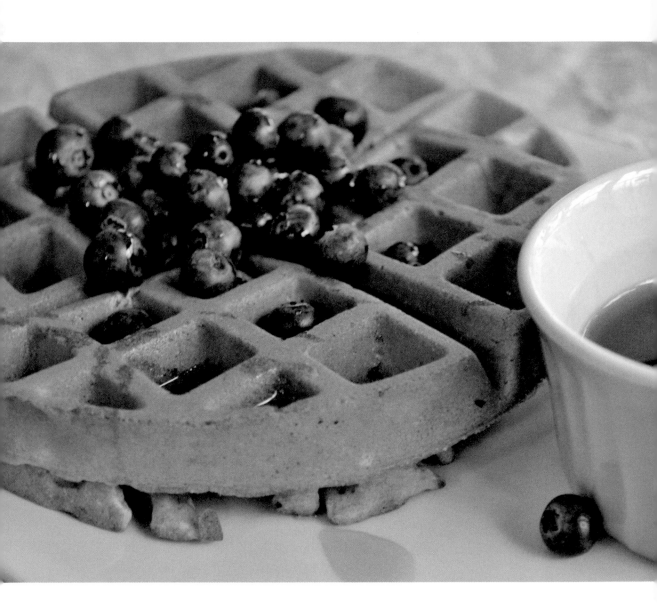

Wild-Rice Waffles

1. Preheat waffle iron according to manufacturer's instructions.

2. In a dry, medium-size bowl, whip egg whites with an electric mixer until stiff peaks form. Set aside.

3. In a separate, large bowl, whisk together flours, baking powder, cinnamon, and salt.

4. In a small bowl, whisk together flaxseed, eggs, milk, oil, and maple syrup. Add the wet ingredients to the dry ingredients. Stir in the cooked wild rice.

5. Fold in the egg whites, one-third at a time, gently incorporating after each addition, being sure to not deflate the egg whites.

6. Grease waffle iron with nonstick cooking spray. Fill waffle maker two-thirds full. Cover and cook about 3 minutes. If you prefer softer waffles, check after 2 minutes. For crispier waffles, cook 1 additional minute.

7. Serve with fresh blueberries and maple syrup. Or serve with Chocolate Syrup NS (page 219), Carob Extract™ (page 249), or Proberry 3™ Liquid (page 250).

2 large egg whites

1 cup brown rice flour

⅓ cup tapioca flour (NS substitute arrowroot starch)

2 teaspoons baking powder

½ teaspoon ground cinnamon (NS omit cinnamon)

¼ teaspoon fine-grain sea salt

1 tablespoon ground flaxseed

2 large eggs

¾ cup almond milk (NS substitute rice milk)

¼ cup vegetable oil

1 tablespoon maple syrup (NS substitute agave)

⅔ cup cooked wild rice

▶ SERVES 4

featured ingredient

flaxseed

Flaxseeds are small with a hard, smooth surface and are packed with omega-3 fatty acids as well as manganese, fiber, and other nutrients. Foods rich in omega-3s are a healthy addition to any diet, and provide anti-inflammatory benefits for Type Os specifically in their ability to fight cancer and diabetes. Flaxseed can be added to smoothies, baked goods, or even used as a topping on salads. When submerged in warm water, flaxseed binds together with the water and forms a gelatin that is helpful in gluten-free baking.

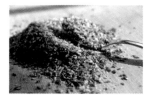

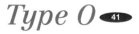

Pumpkin Muffins with Carob Drizzle

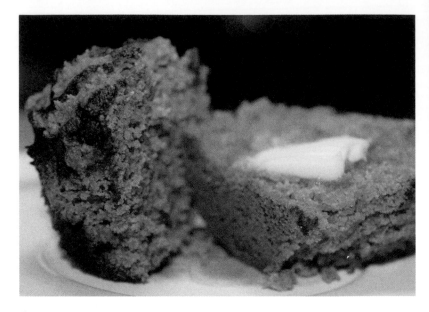

1½ cups brown rice flour

1 cup white rice flour

½ cup tapioca flour (NS substitute arrowroot starch)

2 teaspoons baking powder

½ teaspoon sea salt

½ teaspoon ground cinnamon (NS substitute ⅛ teaspoon allspice)

¼ teaspoon ground ginger

¼ teaspoon ground nutmeg

1 (12-oz.) can organic pumpkin puree

3 large eggs

⅔ cup maple syrup (NS substitute agave)

4 tablespoons ghee, softened

¼ cup Carob Extract™*

1. Preheat oven to 350 degrees. Line a 12-cup muffin tin with paper liners, and set aside.

2. In a large bowl, whisk flours, baking powder, salt, cinnamon, ginger, and nutmeg until well combined.

3. In a separate bowl, whisk pumpkin, eggs, syrup, and ghee. Add pumpkin mixture to flour mixture and stir to incorporate. Spoon batter into prepared muffin tins, and drizzle evenly with Carob Extract™.

4. Bake 20 to 25 minutes, or until a toothpick inserted into muffin comes out clean.

▶ SERVES 12

*Information about purchasing Carob Extract™ can be found in Appendix II: Products (page 249).

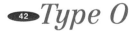

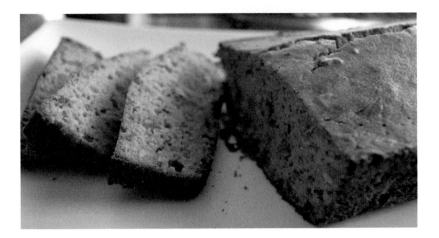

Pear-Rosemary Bread ^{NS}

½ cup diced medium pear

½ cup brown rice flour

¼ cup amaranth flour

¼ cup quinoa flour

1 tablespoon chopped fresh rosemary

½ teaspoon sea salt

2 teaspoons baking powder

3 large eggs, separated

¼ cup agave nectar

¼ cup extra virgin olive oil plus more for greasing

⅓ cup chopped walnuts

1. Preheat oven to 350 degrees. Grease a 5 ½" x 3" loaf pan with olive oil and set aside.

2. Peel and dice pear into small pieces and place on a paper towel to drain excess water.

3. Whisk flours, rosemary, salt, and baking powder to combine, and set aside.

4. In a separate bowl, whisk egg yolks, agave, and olive oil until well combined. Add wet ingredients, pear, and walnuts to dry ingredients, stirring just until mixture is free of lumps.

5. Beat egg whites in a dry, glass bowl until stiff peaks form. Fold into batter, one-third at a time.

6. Spoon batter into prepared loaf pan. Bake 30 to 35 minutes or until cake tester inserted into loaf comes out clean.

7. Serve warm or let cool, place in a resealable glass container, and store in a cool, dry place overnight, or freeze for up to 1 month.

▶ SERVES 10

featured ingredient

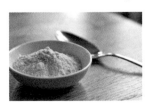

amaranth flour

Amaranth is a gluten-free grain originating from South America. It is high in protein, fiber, and lysine, an amino acid not typically found in grains. Amaranth has a hearty, earthy flavor, and is a great way to add diversity to your diet.

 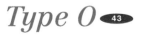

Cherry Scones

½ cup halved dried cherries

1 cup plus 2 tablespoons brown rice flour

¼ cup almond flour

¾ cup white rice flour or tapioca flour

1 tablespoon baking powder

¼ teaspoon baking soda

½ teaspoon sea salt

¼ teaspoon nutmeg

4 tablespoons cold butter or ghee, cubed

½ cup cold maple syrup (NS substitute agave)

¼ cup cold almond milk (NS substitute rice milk)

1 large egg

topping:

1 tablespoon maple syrup (NS substitute agave)

1 tablespoon almond flour

1. Preheat oven to 350 degrees. Line a baking sheet with parchment paper and set aside.

2. Place dried cherries in a small bowl and cover with hot water for 10 minutes to rehydrate. Remove, pat dry, and set aside.

3. In a large mixing bowl, combine flours, baking powder, baking soda, salt, and nutmeg. Stir to combine.

4. Cut butter into the flour mixture using a pastry cutter or by slicing two butter knives until flour resembles coarse cornmeal. Add cherries, mixing just until they are evenly distributed throughout the flour. Set aside.

5. In a separate bowl, whisk maple syrup, milk, and egg until well combined. Fold milk mixture into dry ingredients until well combined. Dough will be thick and slightly lumpy. If necessary, use extra brown rice flour to form the dough into a ball. Gently place on a floured surface, and using your hands, pat dough into a rectangular shape about 1-inch thick. Using a sharp knife, cut the dough horizontally once and then into thirds vertically, to make 6 squares.

6. Cut each square again at an angle to make 12 triangles. Gently place each scone on prepared baking sheet. Brush tops evenly with maple syrup and sprinkle with almond flour.

7. Bake 20 minutes at 350 degrees. Serve warm, or let cool completely and store in a cool, dry place overnight. Scones can be frozen for up to 1 month; reheat in a 200-degree oven for 10 minutes.

▶ SERVES 12

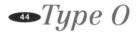

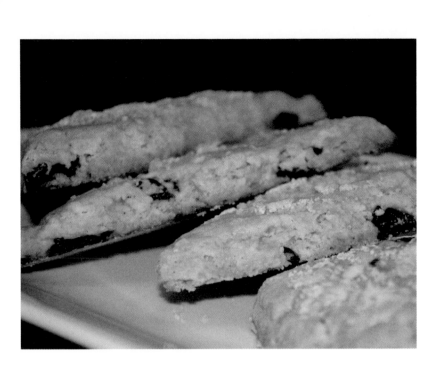

tip: Keeping everything—including your bowls—cold creates a flaky texture in your scones.

featured ingredient

almond flour

To make almond flour, blanched almonds are ground into a fine meal. Almond flour is great to use in baked goods such as cookies, muffins, or dense cakes. It lends a sweet flavor, and adds protein and healthy fats. Almond flour adds a soft grainy texture that helps to make cookies crispier and gives cakes or muffins a hearty, whole-grain feel. For best results, store almond flour in the freezer.

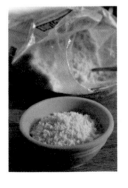

Blueberry-Macadamia Muffins

1 cup brown rice flour

1 cup white rice flour

½ cup millet flour

½ teaspoon sea salt

2 teaspoons baking powder

1 teaspoon baking soda

1 teaspoon cinnamon (NS omit cinnamon)

3 large eggs

⅓ cup agave

⅓ cup honey (NS substitute agave or molasses)

½ teaspoon lemon zest

3 tablespoons light olive oil

6 tablespoons almond milk (NS substitute rice milk)

½ banana

½ cup chopped macadamia nuts

1 cup (fresh or frozen) organic blueberries

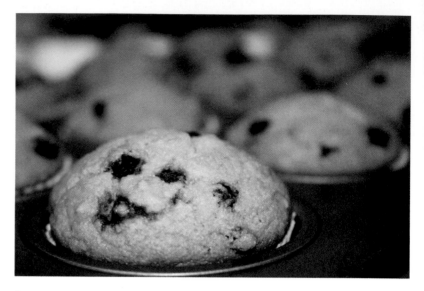

1. Preheat oven to 350 degrees. Line a 12-cup muffin tin with paper liners, and set aside.

2. In a large bowl, combine flours, salt, baking powder, baking soda, and cinnamon. Set aside.

3. In a separate bowl, whisk eggs with agave, honey, lemon zest, olive oil, and almond milk. Mash banana and whisk into egg mixture.

4. Add wet ingredients to dry ingredients, stirring to combine. Fold in macadamia nuts and blueberries. Divide batter evenly among prepared muffin tins and bake for 20 to 25 minutes.

5. Serve warm.

▶ **SERVES 12**

featured ingredient

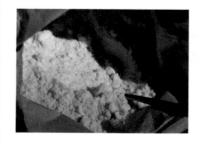

millet flour

Millet is a small, gluten-free grain. A member of the grass family, millet was popular in Africa and India before being introduced in the United States in 1875. Millet is not acid forming so it is easily digested. It has a mild taste and creamy, yellow hue, and is high in fiber, B-complex, and vitamin E, as well as several important minerals.

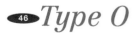 *Type O*

EAT RIGHT FOR YOUR TYPE PERSONALIZED COOKBOOK

Lunch

Adzuki Hummus Sandwich NS ■ *Bacon Grilled Cheese* ■ *Lamb Meatball Subs*
NS ■ *Philly Cheesesteak Sandwich* ■ *Greens and Beans Salad* NS ■ *Salad*
Pizza ■ *Dandelion Greens with Roasted Roots and Horseradish Dressing* NS ■ *Roasted*
Tomato Greek Salad ■ *Salmon-Salad Radicchio Cups* ■ *Baked Falafel* NS ■ *Raw Kale*
Salad with Zesty Lime Dressing NS ■ *Crunchy Kohlrabi Spring Rolls with Sweet Cherry*
Dip NS ■ *Feta, Spinach, and Asparagus Pie* ■ *Ratatouille* NS ■ *White Bean Stew* NS

Each **lunch recipe** is written to provide a balance between vegetables and varying types of proteins while staying lighter on the complex carbohydrates. Recipes that are more dominantly vegetable or protein include suggestions for a tasty complement of the other.

Adzuki Hummus Sandwich NS

2 slices brown rice bread

½ teaspoon olive oil

Large-grain sea salt, to taste

2 tablespoons Adzuki Bean Hummus*

3 thinly sliced rounds green bell pepper

2 leaves Boston Bibb lettuce

1. Toast bread until honey brown, and drizzle one side of each slice with olive oil and a scant sprinkling of sea salt.

2. Spread hummus on the olive oil side of one piece of toast, and top with sliced bell pepper and lettuce leaves. Place the second piece of toast oil side down, and slice in half.

3. Serve immediately.

*See Adzuki Bean Hummus NS recipe (page 167).

▶ SERVES 2

Bacon Grilled Cheese

1 teaspoon olive oil

4 strips turkey bacon

4 teaspoons ghee

4 slices brown rice/millet bread

½ cup shredded mozzarella cheese (NS substitute 2 tablespoons Adzuki Bean Hummus NS and add ¼ cup fresh baby spinach to sandwich)

1. Heat olive oil in a medium skillet set over medium heat. Cook bacon for 1-2 minutes per side. Remove from heat and drain on paper towel.

2. Spread ghee evenly on one side of each piece of bread. Place bacon and cheese on unbuttered side of bread and top with a second piece of buttered bread, so that each outer side of bread is buttered. Toast in a skillet until lightly browned on each side and cheese has melted, about 2 to 3 minute per side.

3. Slice grilled cheese in half and serve with Tomato-Basil Soup NS (page 134).

▶ SERVES 2

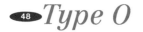

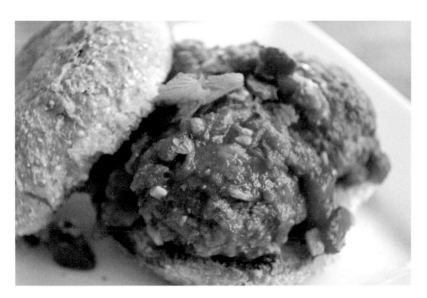

1 pound lean, ground lamb

¼ cup grated onion

⅓ cup finely chopped mint

¼ teaspoon sea salt

1 teaspoon curry powder

1 large egg

5 tablespoons bread crumbs*

sauce:

2 teaspoons olive oil

½ cup chopped onion

2 cups diced red bell pepper

2 cloves garlic, minced

5 vine-ripened tomatoes, chopped

Sea salt, to taste

4 brown rice/millet buns

¼ cup fresh chopped basil, for garnish

1. Preheat oven to 400 degrees. Line a baking sheet with parchment paper and set aside.

2. Place lamb in a large bowl, and add onion, mint, sea salt, curry, egg, and bread crumbs. Gently combine all ingredients with clean hands. Try not to overwork the meat because it will become too tough.

3. Roll meatballs into golf ball–size balls and place on prepared baking sheet about 2 inches apart. Bake for 20 minutes or until golden brown and cooked through.

4. While meatballs cook, prepare tomato sauce. Heat olive oil in a high-sided skillet over medium heat. Once hot, sauté onion, pepper, and garlic for 5 to 6 minutes. Add tomatoes and bring to a boil. Reduce heat, and simmer 10 to 15 minutes. Add salt to taste, and keep warm until ready to serve.

5. Add meatballs to sauce, and toss to coat. Spoon onto buns, and garnish with basil.

6. Serve warm.

*See Basic Gluten-Free Bread Crumbs NS recipe (page 224).

▶ SERVES 4

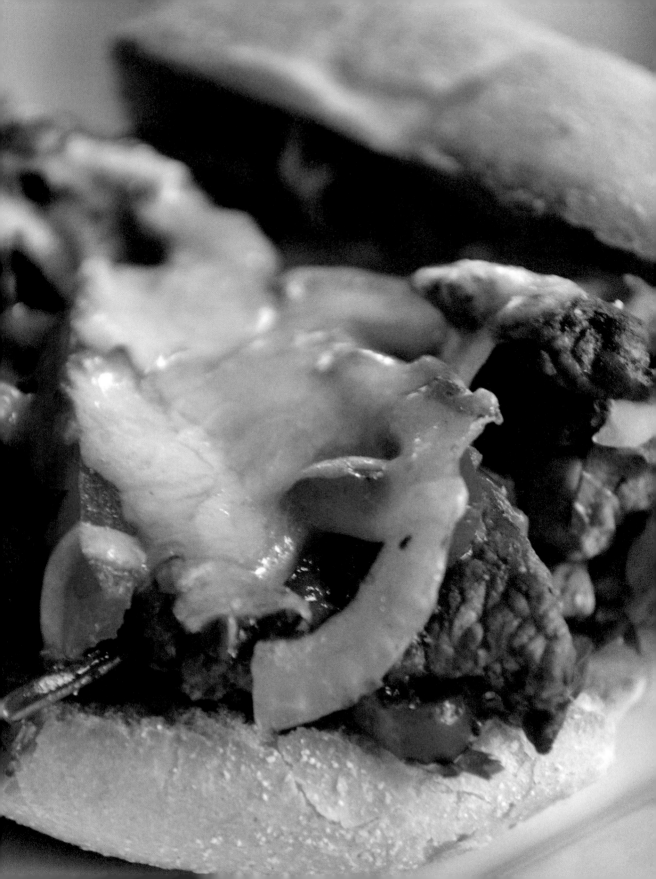

Philly Cheese-steak Sandwich

1. Preheat broiler.

2. Sprinkle sliced beef evenly with cumin, chili, garlic, and sea salt, and use your hands to massage spices into beef.

3. Heat olive oil in a large skillet over medium heat. Once hot, add seasoned steak and sauté 2 to 3 minutes. Remove from heat and set aside.

4. In the same skillet, add peppers and onion. Sauté 8 to 10 minutes, until vegetables are slightly caramelized and tender. Add beef back to the skillet and toss with vegetables.

5. Toast buns and divide mixture evenly among the bottom buns. Top with cheese. Place under broiler for 30 to 60 seconds, just enough to melt the cheese. Top with other halves of buns, and serve warm.

▶ SERVES 4

¾–1 pound lean beef, sliced thin

⅛ teaspoon ground cumin

¼ teaspoon chili powder

¼ teaspoon garlic powder

¼ teaspoon sea salt

2 teaspoons olive oil

1 cup sliced red bell pepper

1 cup sliced green bell pepper

1 cup sliced onions

4 brown rice/millet buns

1 cup part-skim, grated mozzarella cheese (NS substitute manchego cheese or omit cheese)

 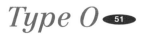

Greens and Beans Salad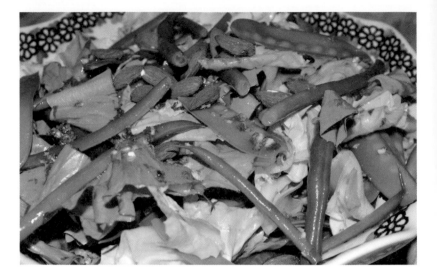

1 head escarole

½ cup canned adzuki beans, drained and rinsed

2 cups snap peas

4 cups string beans

dressing:

1 tablespoon chopped mint

1 tablespoon lime juice

⅛ teaspoon ground cumin

1 clove garlic, minced

½ teaspoon honey (NS substitute agave)

¼ cup olive oil

Sea salt, to taste

1. Wash escarole and pat dry. Tear into bite-size pieces and place into a large serving bowl, top with adzuki beans, and set aside.

2. Bring a large pot of water to a boil. Cook snap peas and string beans for 3 minutes, drain, and transfer to a large bowl of ice water to stop the cooking process. Lay the peas and beans on a kitchen towel to dry, and add to escarole.

3. Whisk together all dressing ingredients in a small bowl. Drizzle over salad and serve.

▶ SERVES 4

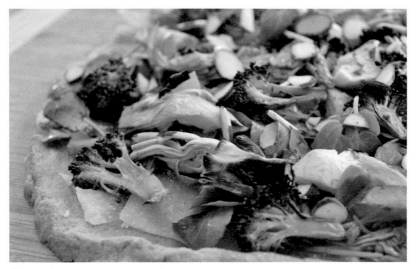

Salad Pizza

1. Preheat oven to 375 degrees.

2. Combine flours, baking powder, and salt. Whisk eggs and olive oil in a small bowl, add to flour mixture, and stir just to combine. Use your hands to form dough into a ball, and roll out on a floured surface until about ¼-inch thick by 9-inches around. Very gently, transfer to a baking sheet and bake for 20 minutes. Remove from oven, layer with goat cheese, and let cool. Increase oven temperature to 400 degrees.

3. Slice artichoke hearts into quarters and pat dry. Cut broccoli into bite-size florets and place on a baking sheet with quartered artichokes. Toss with olive oil and sea salt, and bake for 20 minutes. Remove from oven and set aside.

4. Whisk dressing ingredients together, and toss with watercress, artichokes, broccoli, and almonds. Top crust with salad mixture, and serve cold.

▶ SERVES 4

crust:

⅓ cup quinoa flour

⅓ cup amaranth flour

⅔ cup brown rice flour

2 teaspoons baking powder

½ teaspoon salt

2 eggs

3 tablespoons olive oil

¼ cup shaved, hard goat cheese (NS omit cheese, and drizzle crust with olive oil and large-grain sea salt)

topping:

1 cup frozen artichoke hearts, thawed

1 head broccoli

1 teaspoon olive oil

Sea salt, to taste

2 cups watercress

1 tablespoon blanched slivered almonds

dressing:

1 tablespoon fresh lemon juice

1 teaspoon onion, minced

1 tablespoon olive oil

2 teaspoons fresh oregano, chopped

 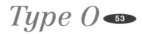

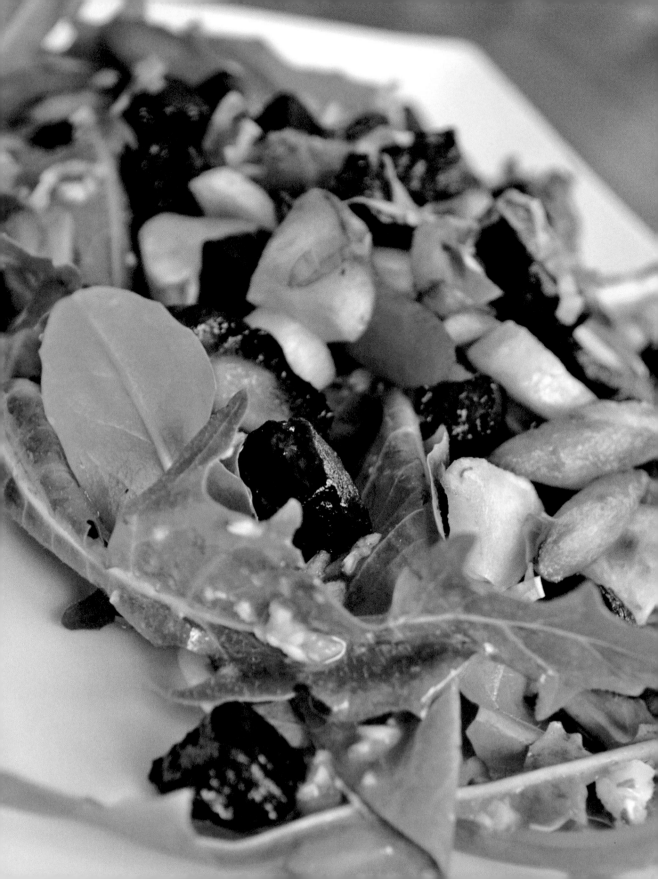

Dandelion Greens with Roasted Roots and Horseradish Dressing (NS)

1. Preheat oven to 375 degrees.

2. Peel beet, carrots, and parsnips. Dice vegetables into ½-inch cubes. Toss with olive oil and season with sea salt. Spread in a single layer on a baking sheet and bake for 55 to 60 minutes, tossing halfway through.

3. To prepare dressing, grate fresh horseradish. Add horseradish to a bowl with olive oil, basil, lemon juice, and sea salt, to taste. Whisk all ingredients to combine.

4. Toss dandelion greens in a large bowl with horseradish dressing, top with roasted vegetables, and serve.

▶ SERVES 4

tip: If you cannot find tricolored carrots, plain carrots will work just fine.

1 raw beet
3 small tricolored carrots
2 medium parsnips
2 teaspoons olive oil
Sea salt, to taste

dressing:
¼ cup fresh, finely grated horseradish
¼ cup olive oil
1 tablespoon fresh basil
2 tablespoons lemon juice
Sea salt, to taste

2 bunches dandelion greens

Roasted Tomato Greek Salad

1 pint heirloom cherry tomatoes

1 teaspoon olive oil

Sea salt, to taste

dressing:

1 tablespoon fresh oregano

2 tablespoons fresh squeezed lemon juice

3 tablespoons olive oil

Sea salt, to taste

6 cups torn romaine lettuce

½ cup Spanish green olives (NS omit olives)

½ cup crumbled feta cheese (NS omit cheese and add 2 chopped green banana peppers to the roasting pan with tomatoes)

1. Preheat oven to 375 degrees.

2. Place tomatoes on a baking sheet. Drizzle with olive oil, sprinkle with sea salt, and bake for 35 minutes on top rack of the oven, until tomatoes collapse and are slightly charred. Remove from oven and let cool.

3. Whisk dressing ingredients together in a small bowl, and set aside.

4. Place lettuce in a serving bowl. Add roasted tomatoes, olives, feta cheese, and dressing, and toss to combine.

▶ SERVES 4

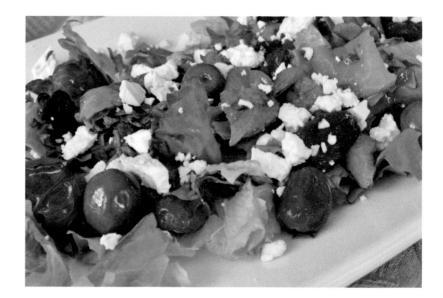

Salmon-Salad Radicchio Cups

1. Peel outer leaves of the radicchio, and discard the first couple of leaves. Continue peeling inner leaves gently, snapping at the base to maintain the integrity of each leaf. Clean with cold water and let dry on a kitchen towel.

2. Flake salmon into a bowl, and add chives, salt, peas, and apples.

3. Whisk together honey, oregano, lemon juice, lime zest, and olive oil in a small bowl. Drizzle over salmon mixture and spoon salmon into cleaned radicchio cups.

▶ **SERVES 2**

1 head radicchio

½ pound salmon, cooked

3 tablespoons diced chives

½ teaspoon sea salt

½ cup cooked peas

½ cup finely diced apples (NS substitute Bosc pear)

1 teaspoon honey (NS substitute agave)

1 teaspoon chopped fresh oregano

Juice of 1 lemon

Zest of 1 lime

¼ cup olive oil

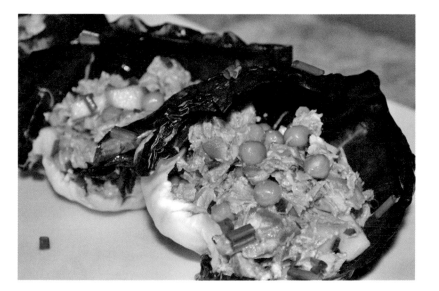

 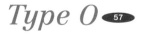

Baked Falafel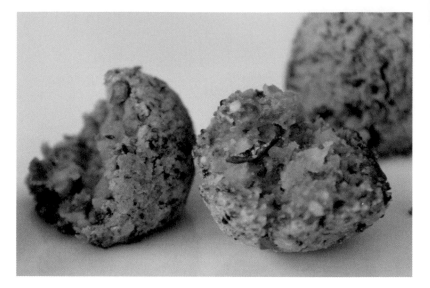

1½ cups soaked adzuki beans (not canned or precooked)

1 tablespoon olive oil, divided

½ cup chopped parsley

2 tablespoons brown rice flour

1 cup chopped onion

2 cloves garlic, minced

¼ teaspoon ground coriander

¼ teaspoon ground cumin

½ teaspoon sea salt

1. Place beans in a pot with enough water to cover by 1-inch, and bring to a boil. Boil for 30 minutes, drain, and rinse. Beans will be slightly firm; this will help falafel's texture. Place beans in a single layer on a paper towel to dry.

2. Preheat oven to 350 degrees. Brush a baking sheet with 1 to 2 teaspoons olive oil, and set aside.

3. In a food processor, add beans, parsley, flour, onion, garlic, coriander, cumin, and salt. Pulse until ingredients form a thick paste. Using a tablespoon measure, roll into a ball and place on prepared baking sheet. Repeat with remaining mixture. Brush remaining olive oil on the tops of falafel and bake for 25 minutes.

4. Increase oven temperature to 400 degrees and bake an additional 15 minutes. Serve on top of Roasted Tomato Greek Salad (page 56).

▶ SERVES 4

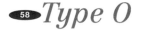

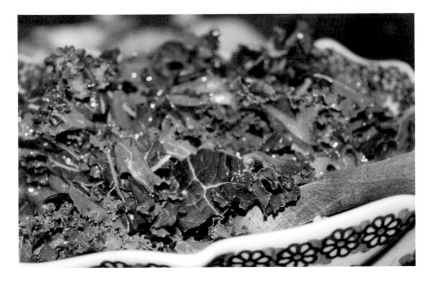

Raw Kale Salad with Zesty Lime Dressing NS

1 bunch kale

2 teaspoons olive oil

1 large white onion, sliced

½ cup raisins

dressing:

2 tablespoons olive oil

Juice of 2 limes

1 clove garlic, minced

⅛ teaspoon ground cumin

Sea salt, to taste

1. Wash kale and dry on kitchen towels. Strip kale off the woody stems by holding the stem with one hand and wrapping finger and thumb of the other hand around the stem and pulling quickly down. Discard stems and tear leaves into bite-size pieces. Place in a large bowl and set aside.

2. Heat olive oil in a skillet over medium heat and sauté onion for 3 to 4 minutes. Add raisins and continue cooking for 5 minutes. Remove from heat and toss with kale.

3. In a small bowl, whisk all dressing ingredients until combined. Drizzle over kale salad and toss to coat.

4. Serve with leftover or chilled baked salmon, roasted chicken, or beans for added protein.

▶ SERVES 6

 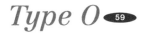

Crunchy Kohlrabi Spring Rolls with Sweet Cherry Dip NS

1 bulb kohlrabi

3 small, tricolored carrots

2 teaspoons olive oil

¼ cup finely chopped onion

¼ cup julienned fresh basil

⅓ cup diced enoki mushrooms

4 large rice paper wraps

1 cup halved cooked medium shrimp (optional)

Sea salt, to taste

sweet cherry dip:

⅓ cup (no sugar added) cherry jam

1 tablespoon fresh grated ginger

1 tablespoon finely diced onion

1 teaspoon agave

Juice of ½ lemon

Sea salt, to taste

1. Prepare kohlrabi by pulling leaves off stalks, then wash and set aside to dry on a kitchen towel. Peel the outer layer of skin off the bulb and slice off tough top and bottom. Slice into thin matchsticks and set aside.

2. Peel and slice carrots into thin matchsticks, and set aside.

3. Heat olive oil in a skillet over medium heat and sauté onion for 5 to 6 minutes. Add kohlrabi greens and sauté 2 minutes, season with sea salt to taste. Remove from heat and let cool.

4. Add carrots, kohlrabi bulb, basil, and enoki mushrooms to sautéed vegetables, and toss to combine.

5. Pour hot water halfway up a large, flat-bottomed bowl. Submerge rice paper wrap in water until it softens and becomes pliable, about 30 seconds. Rice paper is delicate, so be gentle. Place rice wrap on a cutting board and spoon about 2 tablespoons of the vegetable mixture and a few pieces of shrimp (for added protein) down the center of the rice paper. Roll the sides over the vegetables first, and then pull the top over the vegetables and continue to roll. Slice in half, and repeat until remaining rice papers and filling is used.

6. In a small saucepan, combine all sauce ingredients. Warm over low heat for 1 to 2 minutes until warmed through, stirring occasionally.

7. Serve wraps with cherry dip.

▶ SERVES 2

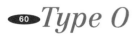

featured ingredient

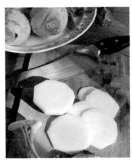

kohlrabi

Crunchy and mildly sweet, the texture of kohlrabi is reminiscent of a Granny Smith apple. Kohlrabi is a member of the cabbage family and is close in taste to broccoli, but more mild and slightly sweet. It looks like a root, but actually grows above ground and is abundant with nutritional value for Type O. The bulb sprouts long stems with leafy tops, which are also edible. Kohlrabi can be eaten raw or cooked.

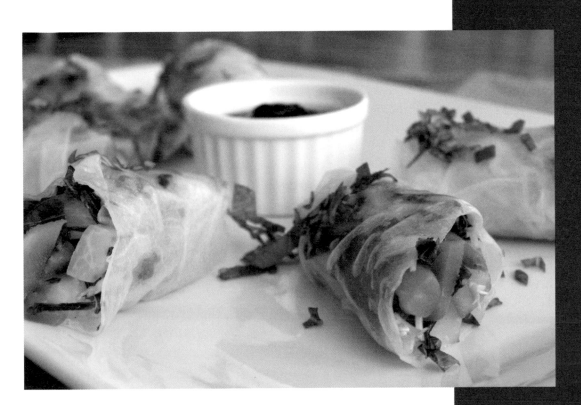

Feta, Spinach, and Asparagus Pie

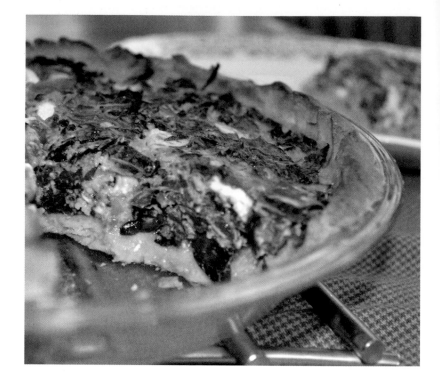

crust:

2 tablespoons quinoa flour

⅓ cup millet flour

⅔ cup brown rice flour

1 teaspoon baking powder

½ teaspoon salt

4 tablespoons cold, unsalted butter or ghee

5 tablespoons ice water

filling:

2 teaspoons olive oil

4 cups baby spinach

2 cups red kale

1 tomato, diced

1 cup sliced asparagus

2 shallots, diced

1 cup crumbled feta cheese (NS omit cheese)

2 large eggs

⅓ cup Vegetable Stock*

2 tablespoons fresh thyme

Sea salt, to taste

1. Preheat oven to 375 degrees.

2. Combine flours, baking powder, and salt in a large bowl. Cut in cold butter with two butter knives or a pastry cutter until flour resembles coarse cornmeal. Add cold water 1 tablespoon at a time, gently incorporating after each addition, just until mixture forms a dough. Flour a surface with brown rice flour, and roll out dough until 12 inches in diameter and ¼ inch thick. Carefully place in a 9-inch pie plate, push down into the sides of the pan, and crimp edges by pinching dough between fingers.

3. Par-bake crust for 15 minutes. ("Par-bake" means that you are partially baking the crust before adding the filling.)

4. While the crust bakes, heat olive oil in a large skillet over medium heat. Sauté spinach, kale, tomato, asparagus, and shallots for 4 minutes, just until vegetables are tender. Remove from heat, place in a large bowl, toss with feta, and set aside to let cool.

5. In a separate bowl, whisk eggs, stock, thyme, and salt. Pour over cooled vegetables and mix to combine.

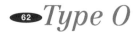
EAT RIGHT FOR YOUR TYPE PERSONALIZED COOKBOOK

6. Pour filling into par-baked pie crust, and bake 30 minutes, or until filling is firm.

7. Serve warm or let cool and refrigerate until cold.

*See Vegetable Stock NS recipe (page 223).

▶ SERVES 6

featured ingredient

quinoa/quinoa flour

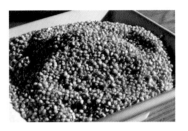

Quinoa is an ancient grain cultivated by the Incan tribes that has only recently regained popularity. It is a fantastic meal in itself because it is high in fiber and contains all nine essential amino acids, making it a complete source of protein. When cooked, quinoa has a slightly nutty flavor and a light, soft texture with a subtle crunch from the outer shell of the grain. It can be used in most recipes as a substitute for rice, or even eaten with dried fruit and nuts for a warm breakfast treat! As an added bonus, quinoa takes only 12 minutes to cook. The grain is also ground into a flour that can be used to make breads, pancakes, biscuits, or other baked goods. Quinoa flour lends a hearty, slightly bitter taste that works well when mixed with other flours such as brown rice or millet. Because of its unique flavor, it also works well in savory baked goods, like cheesy herb biscuits or breadsticks.

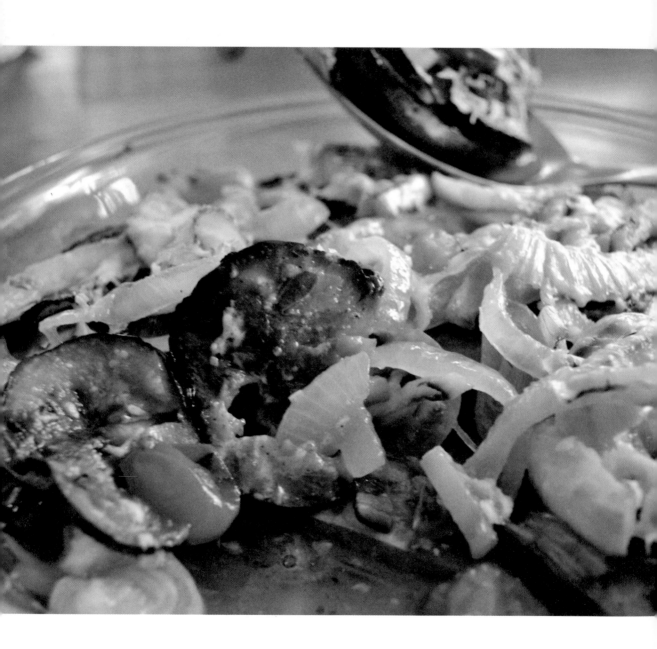

Ratatouille
NS

1. Preheat oven to 375 degrees.

2. Slice eggplant and zucchini into ¼-inch rounds, set on a towel, and sprinkle with sea salt to draw out excess moisture.

3. Slice fennel, tomatoes, and onion into ¼-inch rounds and set aside.

4. Heat 2 teaspoons olive oil in a large skillet over medium heat. Carefully brown fennel and onion in the pan, ensuring vegetables remain in a single layer, 2 to 3 minutes per side. (NS instead of browning artichokes, simply sauté with tomatoes, parsley, and garlic, and proceed with remainder of recipe as written.) Remove from skillet and set aside.

5. Pat excess moisture from eggplant and zucchini slices and brown in the same skillet, 2 to 3 minutes per side, adding additional oil as necessary. Remove from pan and set aside.

6. Sauté tomatoes, parsley, and garlic in pan over medium-high heat for 3 to 4 minutes, allowing some of the liquid from the tomatoes to evaporate.

7. In a glass pie plate or an 8" x 8" baking dish, layer zucchini and eggplant across the bottom, and top with tomato mixture and ¼ cup cheese. Top with onion and fennel and remaining cheese.

8. Bake, uncovered, 20 minutes. Cheese will be caramel brown in color, and vegetables will be wilted and bubbling. Serve warm or cool to room temperature, store in refrigerator, and serve cold.

9. Serve with fresh, sliced mozzarella cheese for added protein. (NS substitute manchego cheese or omit cheese.)

▶ SERVES 4

1 medium eggplant (NS substitute quartered frozen artichokes, thawed and drained)

2 medium zucchini

Sea salt, to taste

1 bulb fennel

2 cups mini heirloom tomatoes

1 large white onion

2 tablespoons olive oil, divided

½ cup chopped parsley

2 cloves garlic

½ cup grated mozzarella (NS substitute manchego cheese or omit cheese)

White Bean Stew NS

2 teaspoons olive oil

1 cup diced onion

1 celery root (celeriac), peeled and diced

2 cups diced orange bell pepper

2 cans organic white beans, drained and rinsed

1½ cups Vegetable Stock*

1 clove garlic

1 sprig sage

4 sprigs thyme

1 teaspoon sea salt

2 cups snow peas

1. In a large Dutch oven, heat olive oil over medium heat. Add diced onion and celery root, and sauté 4 to 5 minutes. Add pepper and sauté an additional 2 to 3 minutes, until vegetables are tender and aromatic.

2. Add beans, stock, garlic, sage, thyme, and salt, and bring to a gentle boil. Reduce heat, cover, and simmer 25 minutes.

3. Add snow peas and cook 5 minutes.

4. Remove sage and thyme and serve warm.

*See Vegetable Stock NS recipe (page 223).

► SERVES 4

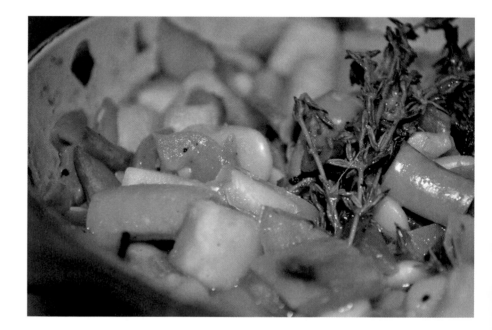

EAT RIGHT FOR YOUR TYPE PERSONALIZED COOKBOOK

Dinner

Roasted Tomato and Broccoli Mac and Cheese ■ Pasta Carbonara with Crispy Kale ■ Spring Pesto Pasta ■ Sweet Potato Gnocchi with Basil-Cranberry Sauce NS ■ Veggie Lasagna ■ Grilled Radicchio and Walnut-Spinach Pesto NS ■ Noodles with Poached Salmon and Creamy Basil Sauce NS ■ Salmon–Black Bean Cakes with Creamy Cilantro Sauce NS ■ Lemon-Ginger Salmon ■ Baked Mahimahi with Crunchy Fennel Salad ■ Parchment-Baked Snapper NS ■ Fig and Basil Halibut NS ■ Spicy Seafood Stew NS ■ Fish Tacos with Sweet Mango-Bean Salad ■ Seafood Paella ■ Fig-Stuffed Turkey Breasts NS ■ Turkey Sausage–Stuffed Peppers NS ■ Turkey-Ginger Stir-Fry NS ■ Hearty Slow-Cooker Turkey Stew NS ■ Turkey Mole Drumsticks ■ Crispy-Coated Turkey Tenderloins with Apricot Dipping Sauce ■ Shredded Turkey Bake ■ Green Tea–Poached Chicken NS ■ Chicken Pot Pie with Crunchy Topping NS ■ Broccolini-Stuffed Chicken ■ Beef Tips with Wild Mushrooms NS ■ Beef and Bean Chili ■ Braised Brisket ■ Tangy Pineapple and Beef Kabobs NS ■ Sweet Potato Shepherd's Pie ■ Sun-Dried Tomato Burgers on Millet Buns NS ■ Grilled Lamb Chops with Mint Pesto NS ■ Moroccan Lamb Tagine ■ Slow-Cooker Venison NS ■ Meat Loaf ■ Red Quinoa–Mushroom Casserole with Fried Eggs NS ■ Sprouted Lentil Stew NS ■ Spaghetti Squash with Goat Cheese and Walnuts

The bulk of the recipes in this book are in this section. Here you will find a variety of dishes, from pastas to seafood to all-in-one dishes. Most of the recipes are simple to make, but others take a bit more time to prepare. Hopefully these dishes inspire you to take some time to enjoy delicious, wholesome food for yourself and your family.

Roasted Tomato and Broccoli Mac and Cheese

1 large head broccoli

4 plum tomatoes

1 tablespoon olive oil

1 tablespoon fresh thyme

Sea salt, to taste

⅔ cup bread crumbs*

1 tablespoon ghee

2 tablespoons white rice flour

2 cups Vegetable Stock*

1 cup almond milk (**NS** substitute rice milk)

1 tablespoon chopped fresh sage

1 pound brown rice or quinoa elbow pasta

1 cup shredded mozzarella cheese

½ cup cubed, fresh mozzarella cheese

1. Preheat oven to 375 degrees.

2. Cut broccoli and tomato into bite-size pieces. Place in a single layer on a baking sheet, drizzle with olive oil, and sprinkle with fresh thyme and sea salt. Bake for 30 minutes. Remove from oven and set aside.

3. Toss bread crumbs with 2 teaspoons of melted ghee and a pinch of sea salt, and set aside.

4. Melt remaining 1 tablespoon ghee in a saucepan over medium heat and whisk in rice flour to form a paste. Gradually add stock and milk to flour mixture, whisking continuously until smooth and free of lumps. Add sage and bring to a boil, whisking constantly. Reduce to a simmer, cooking until the roux thickens, about 10 minutes. Add salt, to taste.

5. Bring a large pot of water to boil, and cook pasta according to package directions. (If using brown rice pasta, cook 8 minutes, slightly less than half of recommended cooking time.) Drain and pour into casserole dish. Toss with roasted vegetables. Pour roux over pasta and top with shredded mozzarella cheese, mixing to incorporate the cheese and sauce. Top with reserved bread crumbs and cubed mozzarella.

6. Bake 20 to 25 minutes. Serve warm.

*See Basic Gluten-Free Bread Crumbs **NS** recipe (page 224). See Vegetable Stock **NS** recipe (page 223).

▶ SERVES 6

Pasta Carbonara with Crispy Kale

1. Bring a large pot of water to boil. Cook pasta 4 minutes less than recommended cooking time.

2. While pasta cooks, heat olive oil in a large, high-sided skillet and sauté onion for 4 to 5 minutes. Add turkey bacon and sauté until browned, 3-4 minutes. Remove turkey bacon and set aside. Add Swiss chard and kale to onion, and sauté until tender, about 3 to 4 minutes. Chop bacon into small, bite-size pieces, add to skillet, and reduce heat to low.

3. Drain pasta, and reserve ½ cup cooking water.

4. In a bowl, whisk together eggs, egg yolks, almond milk, salt, and pepper. Slowly pour pasta cooking water into the egg mixture to temper the eggs. Remove skillet from the heat, add pasta, and slowly add egg mixture. The heat from the pasta will gently cook the eggs and create a sauce.

5. Stir in mozzarella cheese and serve immediately.

▶ SERVES 6

1 pound brown rice pasta

2 teaspoons olive oil

½ cup diced onions

4 slices turkey bacon

3 cups chopped Swiss chard

3 cups chopped red kale

2 large eggs

2 large egg yolks

¼ cup almond milk (NS substitute rice milk)

Sea salt and black pepper, to taste

½ cup pasta water

¼ cup grated mozzarella cheese (NS omit cheese)

 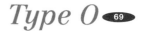

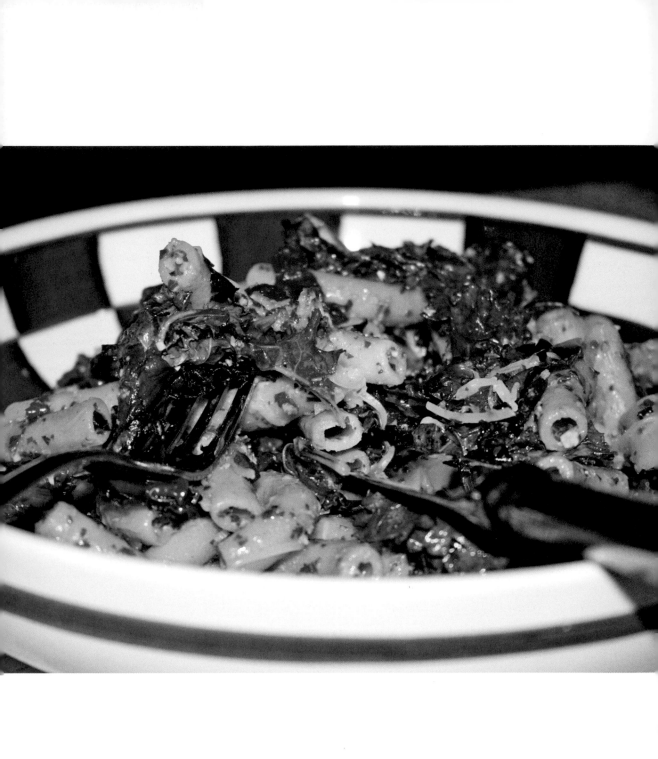

Spring Pesto Pasta

1. Preheat oven to 375 degrees.

2. Snap asparagus spears close to the bottom and discard the woody stems. Cut into bite-size pieces and toss in a large bowl with beet greens. Tear 1½ bunches kale into large, bite-size pieces, and add to bowl. Toss with 2 teaspoons olive oil and a pinch of salt.

3. Place vegetables on a baking sheet and bake for 12 minutes, or until vegetables are tender and kale pieces have slightly crispy edges. Remove from oven and set aside. Reduce oven temperature to 200 degrees.

4. Bring a large pot of water to boil. Cook pasta 4 minutes less than recommended cooking time.

5. While pasta cooks, place remaining ½ bunch kale, ½ cup olive oil, lemon juice, lemon zest, walnuts, garlic, and salt, to taste, in a food processor, pulsing until smooth. Transfer to a bowl and set aside.

6. Heat remaining 1 teaspoon oil in a medium skillet over medium heat. Add bacon and cook until crispy, about 2 minutes per side. (Wrap in a paper towel and keep warm in the oven until ready to serve, to keep the bacon crispy.)

7. Drain pasta, and place in a large pasta bowl. Toss immediately with pesto, peas, and roasted vegetables. Sprinkle with crushed red pepper and goat cheese. Crumble bacon and sprinkle on top of pasta.

▶ SERVES 6

1 bunch asparagus

1 bunch beet greens, chopped

2 large bunches kale, divided

½ cup plus 3 teaspoons olive oil

Sea salt, to taste

1 pound brown rice pasta

Juice and zest of 1 lemon, divided

½ cup walnuts

2 cloves garlic, minced

3 slices turkey bacon

2 cups cooked peas

½ teaspoon crushed red pepper

½ cup goat cheese (NS omit goat cheese)

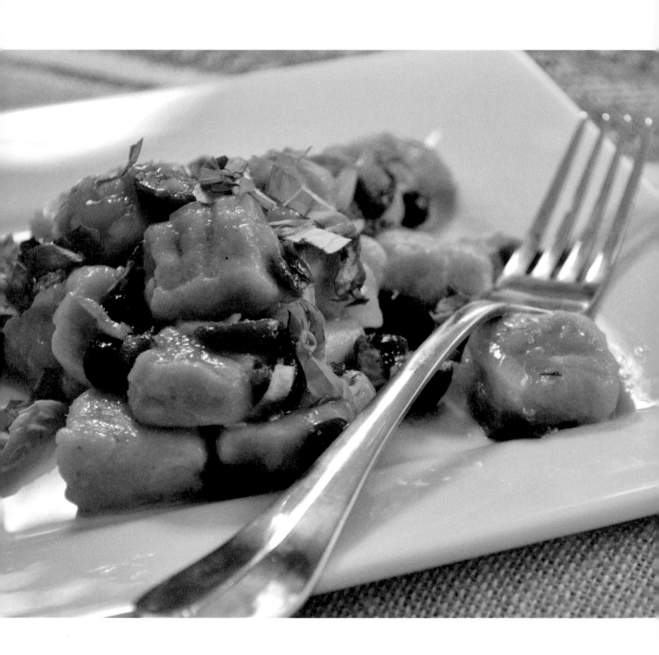

Sweet Potato Gnocchi with Basil-Cranberry Sauce NS

1. Mash boiled sweet potatoes with a fork or potato masher until smooth and creamy.

2. In a large bowl, combine smashed sweet potatoes with remaining gnocchi ingredients. Using your hands, lightly form mixture into a ball. If the dough is too sticky, sprinkle more brown rice flour over the dough. Working with a handful of dough at a time, roll on a floured surface into a long, ¾-inch cylinder. Repeat with remaining dough.

3. Use a sharp knife to slice the cylinders into 1-inch pieces. Roll each piece gently over the back of a fork, to make indentations in the gnocchi.

4. Bring a large pot of salted water to a gentle boil. Add gnocchi in small batches, being careful not to crowd the pot. Gnocchi will float to the top when they are finished cooking, about 2 to 3 minutes. Remove from pot with a slotted spoon, and transfer to a baking sheet until all gnocchi are cooked.

5. While gnocchi cooks, heat olive oil and ghee in a medium skillet over medium heat. Add shallots and sauté 2 to 3 minutes. Add stock, lemon juice, and cranberries.

6. Toss gnocchi with sauce just to coat, garnish with basil, and serve warm.

*See Vegetable Stock NS recipe (page 223).

▶ SERVES 4

2 cups sweet potato, boiled

¾ cup brown rice flour

¼ cup millet flour

1 teaspoon sea salt

1 large egg, beaten

¼ teaspoon fresh ground nutmeg

sauce:

1 tablespoon olive oil

1 teaspoon ghee

¼ cup finely diced shallots

½ cup Vegetable Stock*

1 tablespoon lemon juice

¼ cup dried cranberries

½ cup torn fresh basil

Veggie Lasagna

1 butternut squash

2 large or 3 medium parsnips

2 medium-large Spanish onions

3 tablespoons olive oil, divided

Sea salt, to taste

3 tablespoons butter

4 tablespoons brown rice flour or arrowroot starch

3 cups almond milk (NS substitute rice milk)

¼ cup finely chopped sage

Dash cloves

¼ teaspoon cinnamon (NS omit cinnamon)

2 cloves garlic, minced, divided

1 box brown rice gluten-free lasagna noodles

16 ounces fresh baby spinach

1 cup shredded mozzarella cheese (NS substitute grated manchego cheese)

1. Preheat oven to 400 degrees.

2. Cut off the ends of butternut squash to create a stable base, and peel squash. Cut in half from the base to stem and remove seeds with a spoon. Place the squash, cut side down, on a cutting board and slice into ¼-inch-thick half moons. Peel parsnips and slice on the bias into ¼-inch pieces, and set aside. Peel and slice onions into ¼-inch-thick rings.

3. Place all vegetables in a single layer on baking sheets (you will need 3 sheets), and drizzle each sheet with 2 teaspoons olive oil and sprinkle with sea salt.

4. Bake 25 to 30 minutes, flipping once halfway through. Remove from oven and set aside. Reduce oven temperature to 350 degrees.

5. Melt butter in a large saucepan over medium heat, and add flour, whisking until it forms a paste. Gradually add milk, whisking continuously to prevent lumps. Add sage, cloves, and cinnamon, and 1 clove minced garlic. Whisk until the mixture thickens to the consistency of thin yogurt, 5 to 8 minutes. Remove from heat and set aside.

6. Bring a large pot of water to a boil. Add noodles and cook 5 to 6 minutes, drain, and set aside.

7. Heat 3 teaspoons olive oil in a large skillet over medium heat. Sauté spinach with remaining minced garlic until wilted. Remove from heat and set aside.

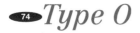 *Type O*

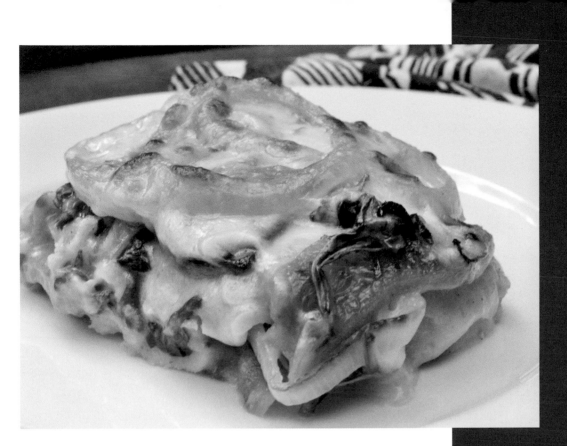

8. Spread a thin layer of sauce in the bottom of a 9" x 11" baking dish. Layer 3 lasagna noodles over sauce and top with one-third of the sauce, roasted parsnips, half the roasted onions, and half the spinach. Top with ½ cup mozzarella cheese. Top with remaining lasagna noodles, one-third of the sauce, butternut squash, remaining spinach, and remaining onions. Pour remaining sauce over lasagna and top with remaining ½ cup mozzarella cheese.

9. Bake lasagna for 20 to 25 minutes, until cheese is melted and bubbling.

10. Serve warm.

▶ **SERVES 6**

DINNER

Grilled Radicchio and Walnut-Spinach Pesto (NS)

infused oil:

Zest of ½ lemon

⅓ cup olive oil

⅛ teaspoon mustard powder

½ teaspoon cumin seeds

2 cloves garlic, smashed

pesto:

¼ cup toasted almonds

2 tablespoons olive oil

2 tablespoons chopped fresh sage

1 cup chopped spinach

2 tablespoons lemon juice

I teaspoon fresh lemon zest

½ teaspoon sea salt

1 tablespoon water

¾ pound spinach brown rice pasta

2 heads radicchio

2 tablespoons toasted almonds

1. In a small skillet, heat all infused oil ingredients over low heat for 15 minutes. Remove from heat and set aside.

2. In a food processor or mini chopper, combine all pesto ingredients. Pulse until mixture is pureed and resembles a thick sauce.

3. Bring a large pot of water to boil. Cook pasta 4 minutes short of recommended cooking time.

4. While the pasta cooks, heat grill pan over medium heat, and brush with infused oil. Peel and discard outer layers of radicchio, then cut radicchio in quarters. Brush each quarter with infused olive oil, and grill about 1 minute per side or until radicchio is tender and slightly wilted.

5. Drain pasta and toss with pesto in a large serving bowl. Top with grilled radicchio and toasted almonds.

6. Serve immediately.

▶ SERVES 4

tip: Reserve remaining infused oil in an oil dispenser and keep in a cool, dry place for up to 2 weeks. Oil is delicious on salads or used as a marinade.

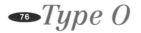

1. Fill a high-sided skillet with stock, water, and lemon slices. Bring to a simmer and add salmon. Cover and cook 12 to 15 minutes.

2. In the meantime, bring a large pot of water to boil. Cook pasta for 4 minutes less than recommended cooking time.

3. While pasta and salmon cook, puree sauce ingredients in a food processor or blender.

4. Drain pasta and toss with all but ¼ cup of the basil sauce. Top with salmon and drizzle with remaining sauce.

5. Serve immediately.

*See Vegetable Stock NS recipe (page 223).

▶ SERVES 4

Noodles with Poached Salmon and Creamy Basil Sauce NS

2 cups Vegetable Stock*
2 cups water
1 lemon, sliced
1½ pounds salmon
¾ pound brown rice pasta

sauce:
2 cups spinach
½ cup Vegetable Stock*
1 cup basil
1 clove garlic, minced
1 cup cooked white beans
2 teaspoons lemon zest
1 teaspoon granulated mustard

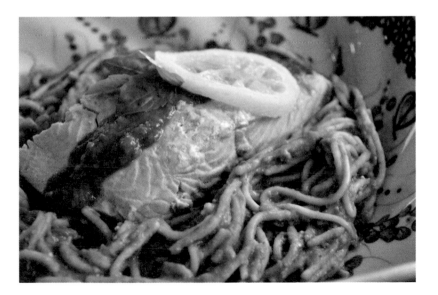

 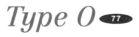

Salmon–Black Bean Cakes with Creamy Cilantro Sauce NS

1 pound wild salmon, cooked

1 cup cooked black beans, drained and rinsed

1 teaspoon chopped scallions

1 teaspoon fresh chopped rosemary

1 teaspoon fresh thyme

Sea salt, to taste

1 large egg, slightly beaten

½ cup bread crumbs*

2 teaspoons olive oil

sauce:

2 tablespoons walnuts

2 tablespoons olive oil

¼ cup cilantro

Sea salt, to taste

1. Flake cooked salmon into a bowl, and carefully remove any bones. Add beans, scallions, rosemary, thyme, and salt. Gently stir in egg and bread crumbs.

2. Heat olive oil in a large skillet over medium heat. Form salmon mixture into patties. Cook 3 to 4 minutes, turn, and cook an additional 3 to 4 minutes on the opposite side.

3. In a food processor, chop walnuts until they form a paste. With processor running add olive oil through feed tube. Once creamy, add cilantro and salt.

4. Serve salmon cakes warm, drizzled with cilantro sauce.

*See Basic Gluten-Free Bread Crumbs NS recipe (page 224).

▶ SERVES 4

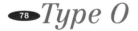

Lemon-Ginger Salmon

1. Preheat oven to 400 degrees.

2. Rub salmon with 1 teaspoon olive oil and season with sea salt.

3. In a small bowl, mix lemon zest, lemon juice, remaining 1 teaspoon olive oil, ginger, and honey until combined. Brush evenly over the top of salmon.

4. Bake for 10 to 12 minutes.

5. Serve with Grilled Sesame-Ginger Bok Choy (page 138).

▶ SERVES 2

1 pound wild salmon fillets

2 teaspoons olive oil, divided

½ teaspoon sea salt

Zest of 1 lemon

1 tablespoon lemon juice

2 tablespoons grated ginger

1 teaspoon honey (NS substitute agave)

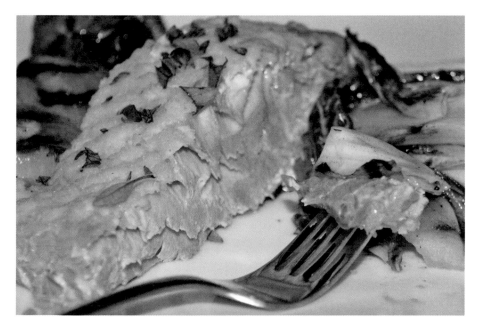

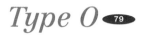

Baked Mahimahi with Crunchy Fennel Salad

1 pound mahimahi

⅛ teaspoon ground coriander

1 teaspoon fresh lemon zest

¼ teaspoon sea salt plus more to taste

2 teaspoons chopped parsley

2 teaspoons olive oil

1 teaspoon lemon zest

2 teaspoons lemon juice

2 cups thinly sliced fennel

1 cup thinly sliced Granny Smith apple (NS substitute sliced plums)

1. Preheat oven to 350 degrees.

2. Season mahimahi with coriander, lemon zest, and ¼ teaspoon sea salt. Bake for 12 to 15 minutes, or until fish is flaky and white.

3. While fish bakes, whisk together parsley, olive oil, sea salt, to taste, lemon zest, and juice in a bowl. Add fennel and apple, and toss to combine.

4. Plate fish, top with fennel salad, and serve immediately.

▶ SERVES 2

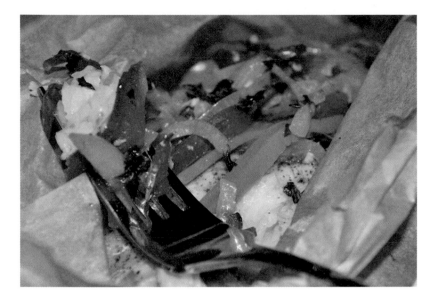

Parchment-Baked Snapper NS

1 pound snapper (4 fillets)

½ teaspoon sea salt

½ teaspoon chili powder

2 cloves garlic, minced

1 cup thinly sliced peaches

1 cup thinly sliced plum tomatoes

1 cup thinly sliced red onion

½ cup sliced orange bell peppers

1 tablespoon plus 1 teaspoon olive oil

1. Preheat oven to 350 degrees.

2. Cut 4 pieces of parchment paper into 12 to 15-inch sections. Fold parchment pieces in half and cut into a large heart shape, like cutting out a valentine. Place 1 snapper fillet in one half of the parchment heart, and repeat with remaining fillets and parchment hearts. Season with salt, chili powder, and garlic.

3. Top snapper with peaches, plum tomatoes, onion, and bell peppers and drizzle each fillet with 1 teaspoon olive oil.

4. Wrap fish in parchment paper by folding edges over. Start at the top of the heart to roll and crease the edges, and crimp ends of parchment paper to seal the sides. Place hearts on a baking sheet and bake for 12 to 15 minutes or until snapper is flaky, opaque, and can be easily flaked with a fork.

5. Serve warm.

▶ SERVES 4

 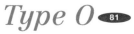

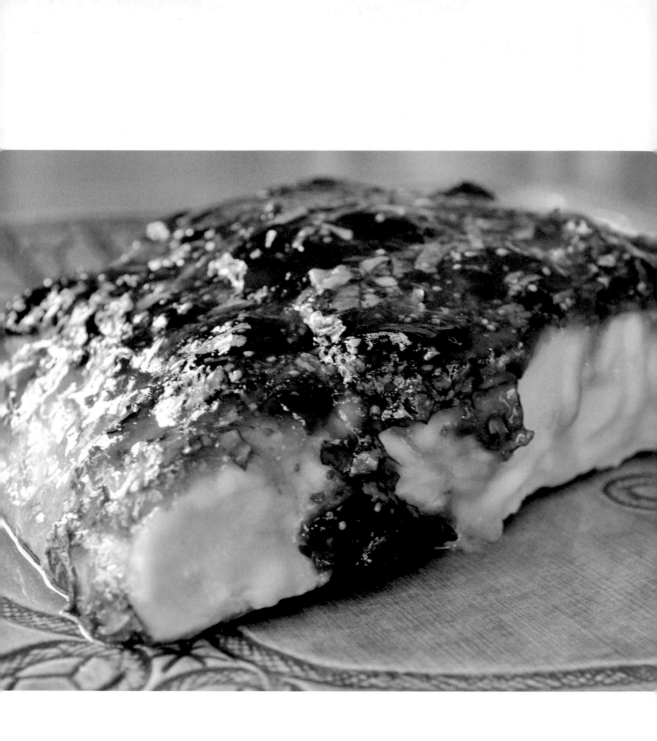

1. Preheat oven to 400 degrees.

2. Slice halibut into 2 fillets.

3. Drizzle halibut with olive oil and sea salt.

4. In a small bowl, whisk fig jam, basil, lemon zest, and lemon juice to combine. Spread evenly over top of halibut, and place in a baking dish.

5. Bake for 30 minutes or until center of fish is flaky and opaque.

▶ SERVES 4

1 pound wild halibut steak

1 teaspoon olive oil

½ teaspoon sea salt

¼ cup fig jam

2 tablespoons chopped fresh basil

2 teaspoons lemon zest

1 teaspoon lemon juice

Spicy Seafood Stew NS

1–2 dried ancho chili peppers

¼ cup wakame

2 teaspoons olive oil

1 cup diced onions

1 bulb diced fennel

1 red bell pepper, diced

1 jalapeno, finely diced

½ teaspoon turmeric

½ teaspoon fennel seeds

¼ cup tomato paste

Sea salt, to taste

2 (6½-oz.) cans pimientos

2 bay leaves

2 cups Vegetable Stock*

2 cups water

¾ pound cod

½ pound wild-caught salmon

1. Place dried ancho chilies in a small bowl of hot water for 10 to 12 minutes (use smaller amount for less spice). Place wakame in a small bowl of cold water for 10 minutes.

2. Heat olive oil in a stockpot over medium heat, and sauté onion and fennel for 4 to 5 minutes. Add red bell pepper and jalapeno, and sauté an additional 3 to 4 minutes. Season with turmeric, fennel seeds, tomato paste, and salt.

3. Drain wakame, rinse, and immediately add to stew.

4. Drain cans of pimiento and pat dry. Drain chilies and remove stems and seeds. Puree pimiento and chilies in a food processor until very smooth.

5. Add puree, bay leaves, stock, and water to stockpot, and simmer 30 minutes.

6. While the stew simmers, dice cod and salmon into bite-size pieces. Add the seafood to stew and cook an additional 10 minutes or until seafood is cooked through.

7. Serve warm.

*See Vegetable Stock NS recipe (page 223).

▶ SERVES 4

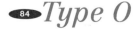
EAT RIGHT FOR YOUR TYPE PERSONALIZED COOKBOOK

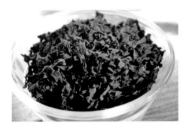

featured ingredient

wakame

If you've had miso soup, you've most likely eaten wakame. Wakame is a nutrient-rich seaweed cultivated off the coast of Japan, and adds a briny finish to soups, stews, and even salads. It is most often dehydrated (as pictured) for distribution, but once soaked, returns to its dark-green color and velvety texture. Seaweed is a *Beneficial* food for Type O, due to its abilities to detoxify the liver. Wakame's mild flavor is a perfect way to begin adding seaweed to your diet.

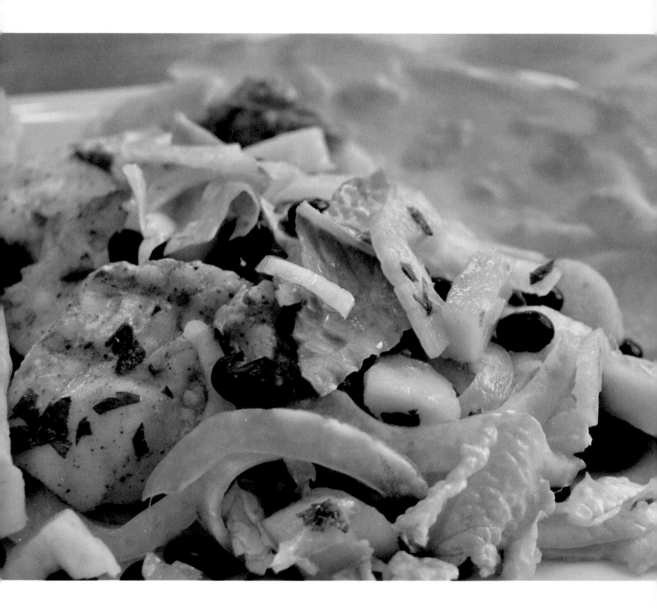

Fish Tacos with Sweet Mango-Bean Salad

1. Combine chili powder, cumin, salt, paprika, and 1 tablespoon olive oil in a small bowl. Slice fish into 1-inch cubes and drizzle spice mixture over fish. Marinate in the refrigerator while preparing the rest of the dish, or at least 20 minutes.

2. Peel rind and pith off the lime and take a paring knife (small sharp knife) to cut the flesh of the lime out from between the membranes, so the sections of lime pop out not surrounded by the fruit's membrane. Place lime sections and all remaining salad ingredients in a large bowl and toss to combine. Set aside while preparing rest of the dish to enable flavors to combine and textures to soften slightly.

3. Whisk all crêpe ingredients together in a large bowl. Heat a large skillet or crêpe pan over medium to medium-high heat. (If not using a nonstick pan, use a nonstick cooking spray.) Using a ¼-cup measure, spoon crêpe batter into skillet, and quickly turn to spread batter into a very thin layer. Let cook about 1 minute, or until the edges start to pull away from the skillet and tiny bubbles appear in the center of the crêpe. Using a large, flat spatula or carefully lifting edges with your hands, flip the crêpe and cook 1 additional minute. Stack crêpes on a plate and keep warm until serving.

4. Heat grill pan over medium heat and brush with remaining 1 teaspoon olive oil. Grill fish 2 to 3 minutes per side, until fish is flaky and opaque.

5. To assemble tacos, place taco crêpe on a plate, and top with fish and fennel slaw.

6. Serve immediately.

▶ SERVES 4

¼ teaspoon chili powder

⅛ teaspoon cumin

½ teaspoon salt

¼ teaspoon paprika

1 tablespoon plus 1 teaspoon olive oil, divided

1 pound swordfish or other whitefish

mango salad:

1 finely sliced fennel bulb

1 tablespoon chopped fresh mint

¼ teaspoon lime zest

1 lime

2 teaspoons olive oil

½ cup diced mango

½ cup cooked black beans, drained and rinsed

¼ teaspoon sea salt

taco crêpes:

2 eggs

½ teaspoon sea salt

⅔ cup brown rice flour

2 tablespoons arrowroot starch

⅓ cup millet flour

1 tablespoon olive oil

1½ cups almond milk (NS substitute rice milk)

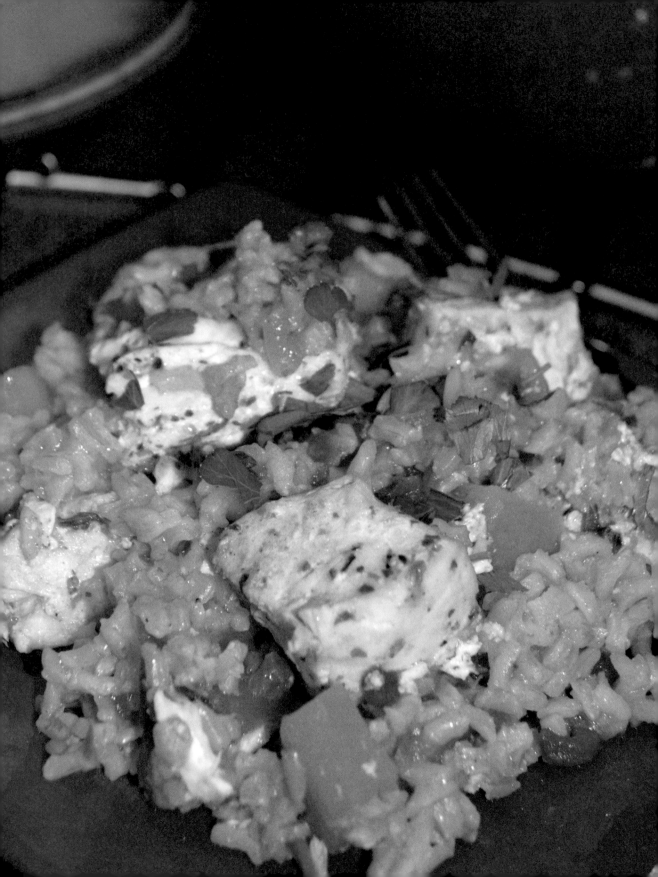

Seafood Paella

1. Preheat oven to 350 degrees.

2. Heat 1 teaspoon olive oil in a large Dutch oven or paella pan over medium heat, and sauté onion and rutabaga for 6 to 7 minutes. Remove vegetables and set aside. Add 1 additional teaspoon olive oil to pan and sauté tomatoes, parsley, jalapeno, and garlic for 4 to 5 minutes. Remove from pan and set aside.

3. Add remaining 1 teaspoon olive oil to same pan and toast brown rice for 2 minutes, stirring continuously. Add saffron, sea salt, and paprika.

4. Return all vegetables to pan, and stir to combine. Add stock, water, bay leaf, and fresh oregano. Bring to a simmer and cover. Place in oven, and bake for 40 minutes.

5. Dice halibut and cod into 1-inch pieces. Toss fish and shrimp in separate bowls with ½ of the dried oregano and sea salt to taste in each.

6. Remove paella from oven and add halibut and cod. Cover and place back in the oven and cook for 7 minutes. Add shrimp and cook an additional 5 minutes. Seafood should be flaky and opaque when fully cooked. Rice will be fluffy and tender.

7. Serve warm.

*See Vegetable Stock NS recipe (page 223).

▶ SERVES 6

3 teaspoons olive oil, divided

2 cups finely chopped yellow onion

1 cup peeled, diced rutabaga

2 vine-ripened tomatoes, chopped

¼ cup chopped parsley

1 jalapeno, diced

2 teaspoons garlic, minced

1½ cups long-grain brown rice

15 threads saffron

1 teaspoon sea salt

1 teaspoon paprika

2 cups Vegetable Stock*

1 cup water

1 bay leaf

2 teaspoons fresh oregano

¾ pound halibut fillets

¾ pound cod fillets

½ pound large shrimp

1 teaspoon dried oregano

Type O 89

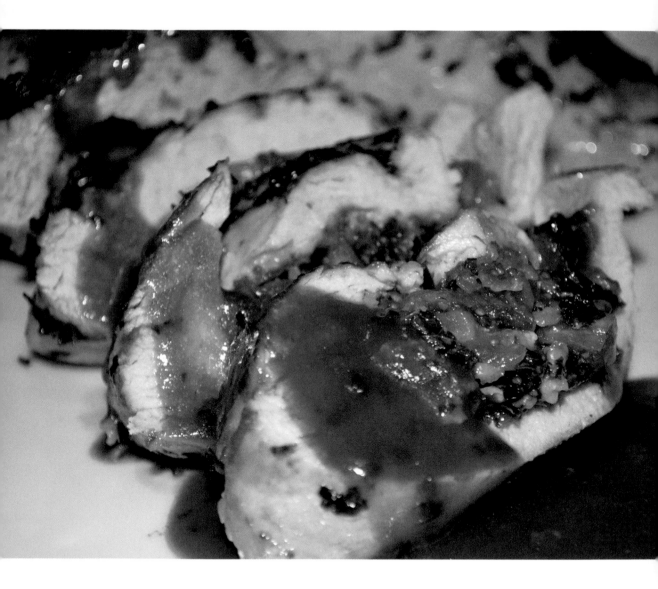

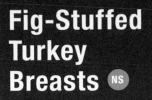
1. Preheat oven to 350 degrees.

2. Finely chop oregano, thyme, and basil, and place in a small bowl. Set aside.

3. Heat 2 teaspoons olive oil and 1 teaspoon ghee in a skillet over medium heat, and sauté shallots for 2 to 3 minutes. Add figs and kale and sauté an additional 4 to 5 minutes. Remove from heat and set aside.

4. Slice turkey breast in half to create two pieces. Butterfly breasts by placing on a cutting board and carefully slicing horizontally through the meat, leaving a ½-inch border. This opens the breast so that stuffing it is made simple. Divide kale stuffing evenly between turkey breasts. Gently pull the turkey back together and fasten with toothpicks. Sprinkle both sides of the stuffed turkey breasts with reserved herb mixture.

5. Heat remaining 1 teaspoon olive oil in an oven-safe skillet over medium heat. Sear stuffed turkey breasts 3 to 4 minutes per side. Transfer skillet to oven and bake for 8 to 10 minutes, or until juices run clear and the internal temperature of the turkey reaches 165 degrees.

6. Remove turkey from pan and place on a cutting board to rest. Place skillet over medium heat and add remaining 1 tablespoon ghee and flour, whisking into a paste. Slowly add stock, whisking continuously to form a gravy. Bring to a simmer and cook 2 to 3 minutes, until the gravy coats the back of a spoon.

7. Slice turkey breast, drizzle with gravy, and serve warm.

*See Turkey Stock NS recipe (page 221). See Vegetable Stock NS recipe (page 223).

Ingredients

1 tablespoon fresh oregano

2 tablespoons fresh thyme

2 tablespoons fresh basil

½ cup shallots, minced

1 tablespoon olive oil, divided

1 teaspoon plus 1 tablespoon ghee or butter

¾ cup chopped figs

2 cups chopped kale

1 large, boneless turkey breast

1 tablespoon brown rice flour

1 cup Turkey or Vegetable Stock*

▶ SERVES 4

 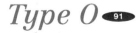

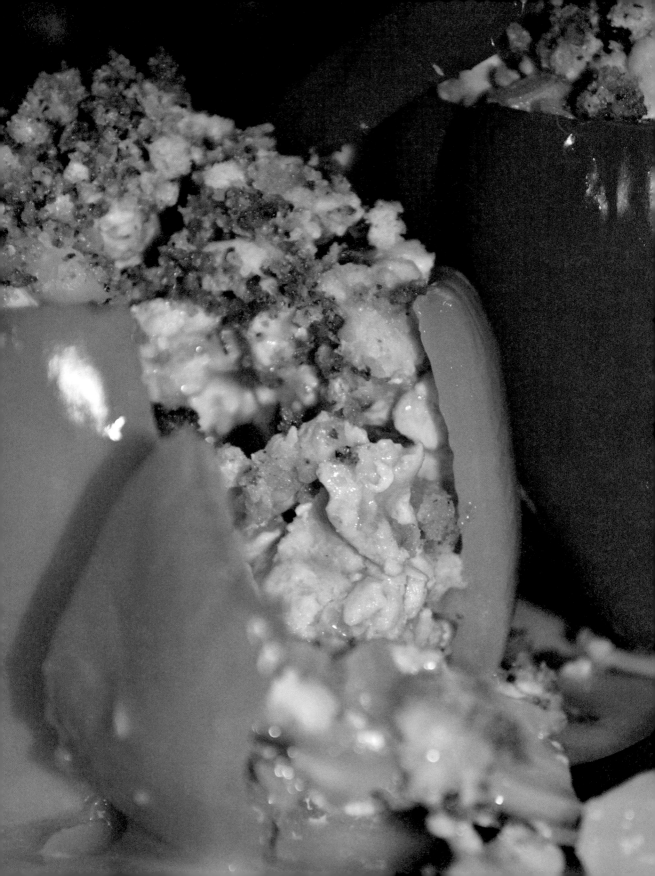

Turkey Sausage– Stuffed Peppers (NS)

1. Preheat oven to 400 degrees.

2. Slice tops off bell peppers to remove the stem. Remove core and seeds, and pat dry. Set peppers and tops on a baking sheet and bake for 20 minutes, until peppers become tender but maintain their shape and the skin is slightly blistered. Remove from oven and set aside.

3. Heat 1 tablespoon olive oil in a large skillet over medium heat. Add fennel seeds, garlic, and mustard powder, and cook for 30 seconds to a minute, to bring out the flavors. Stir continuously to prevent burning. Add onion and fennel, and sauté 4 minutes. Add ground turkey and cook until browned, breaking apart large pieces with a flat, wooden spoon. Add tomatoes, stock, and thyme, and cook another 5 to 6 minutes or until turkey is cooked through. Add brown rice flour, and stir until evenly distributed. Bring to a boil, reduce heat, and simmer for 2 to 3 minutes, until sauce is thickened.

4. Divide turkey mixture evenly among roasted bell peppers, top with bread crumbs, and drizzle 1 teaspoon olive oil over each. Bake 12 minutes or until mixtures is steaming hot and bread crumbs are golden brown.

*See Vegetable Stock NS recipe (page 223). See Basic Gluten-Free Bread Crumbs NS recipe (page 224).

▶ SERVES 4

- 4 bell peppers
- 2 tablespoons plus 1 teaspoon olive oil, divided
- 1 teaspoon fennel seeds
- 2 cloves garlic
- ¼ teaspoon mustard powder
- 1 cup diced onion
- 1 bulb fennel, diced
- 1 pound lean ground turkey
- 2 cups chopped tomatoes
- ½ cup Vegetable Stock*
- 1 tablespoon fresh thyme
- 2 tablespoons brown rice flour
- 1 cup bread crumbs*

Turkey-Ginger Stir-Fry (NS)

3 teaspoons olive oil, divided

1 (2-inch) piece ginger, peeled and thinly sliced

1 pound turkey tenderloins, thinly sliced

2 cups snow peas

1 cup sliced bok choy

¼ cup bamboo shoots

⅓ cup unsweetened plum jam

1 tablespoon lemon juice

1 tablespoon lemon zest

1 tablespoon agave

1. In a large wok or sauté pan, heat 2 teaspoons olive oil over medium heat. Add ginger and sauté 1 minute. Add turkey tenderloins, and stir-fry until cooked, about 3 to 4 minutes. Remove from wok, and set aside.

2. Add remaining olive oil, snow peas, bok choy, and bamboo. Stir-fry 3 to 4 minutes. Return turkey to the wok along with remaining ingredients. Toss to coat and cook 2 additional minutes.

3. Serve hot.

▶ SERVES 4

tip: Bamboo shoots are most commonly found in cans, in the ethnic aisle at the grocery store or natural food market. Rinse bamboo shoots and pat dry before cooking.

2 teaspoons olive oil

1 pound turkey breast

2 cups diced onion

2 cups diced parsnips

2 large sprigs fresh rosemary

4 large sprigs fresh thyme

1 cup water

1 cup Vegetable Stock*

4 cups red kale, torn

1. Preheat slow cooker to medium heat.

2. Heat olive oil in a large skillet over medium heat, and brown turkey breast on all sides. Remove turkey from the pan and set aside.

3. In the same skillet, add onion and parsnips, sautéing 3 to 4 minutes. Add vegetables to the bottom of the slow cooker. Place turkey breast on top of vegetables, then add rosemary and thyme.

4. Pour water and stock in the bottom of the skillet to deglaze, scraping up all the bits. Pour liquid and bits over turkey in the slow cooker and cover.

5. Let cook 1 hour, then add the kale and cook 1 additional hour.

6. Serve warm.

*See Vegetable Stock NS recipe (page 223).

▶ SERVES 4

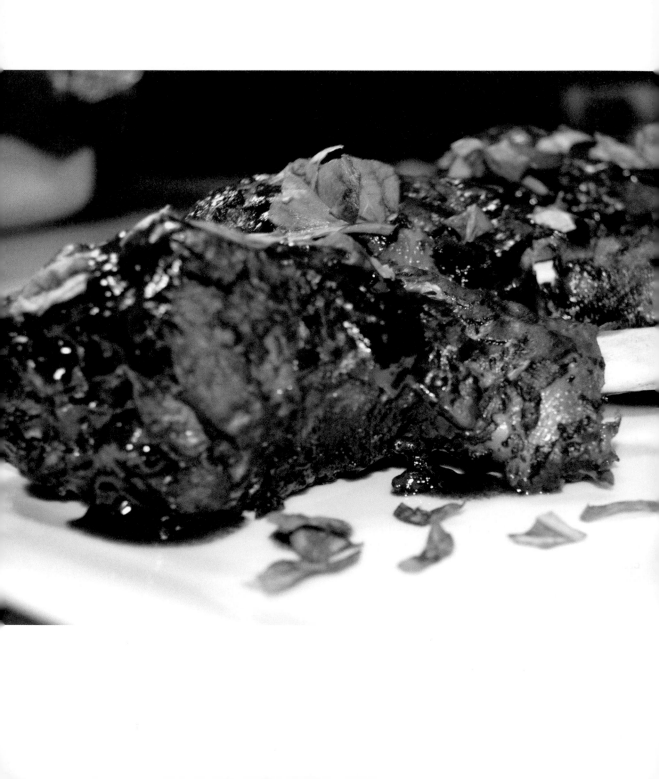

1. Preheat oven to 325 degrees.

2. Melt ghee in a saucepan over medium heat. Sauté garlic and onion for 4 to 5 minutes, until tender and slightly browned. Add cumin, sea salt, chili powder, and cinnamon. Stir and cook an additional 2 minutes. Add tomatoes, stock, and almond butter, stir to combine, and cook 3 to 4 minutes.

3. Remove from heat, stir in chocolate, and transfer to a food processor. Puree until smooth. As an optional step, push mole sauce through a strainer for a silky-smooth sauce.

4. Set aside one-third of sauce. Remove skin from turkey drumsticks and coat with remaining mole sauce. Place in a baking dish, cover and bake for 1 to 1½ hours, until internal temperature reaches 165 degrees.

5. Remove from oven and serve warm, topped with reserved mole sauce.

*See Vegetable Stock NS recipe (page 223).

▶ SERVES 2

1 teaspoon ghee

2 cloves garlic, minced

¼ cup diced onion

1 teaspoon ground cumin

1 teaspoon sea salt

2 teaspoons ancho chili powder

½ teaspoon ground cinnamon (NS omit cinnamon)

1½ cups diced vine-ripened tomatoes

¼ cup Vegetable Stock*

2 teaspoons almond butter

1 ounce 100 percent dark chocolate, shaved

3 turkey drumsticks

tip: Chicken drumsticks can be used in this recipe, but preheat oven to 400 degrees and bake for 50 to 55 minutes, until juices run clear and internal temperature of drumsticks reaches 165 degrees.

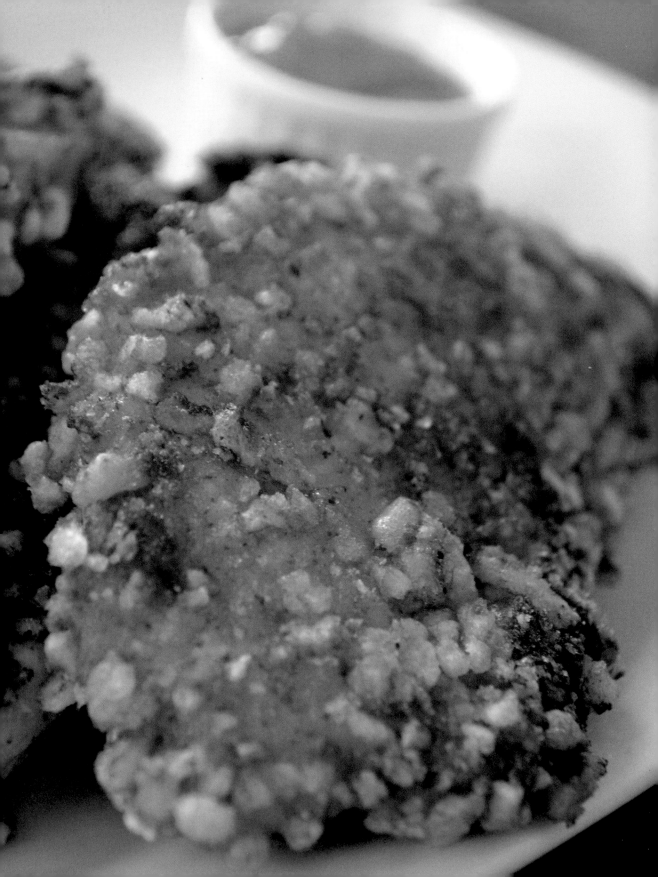

Crispy-Coated Turkey Tenderloins with Apricot Dipping Sauce

1. Grind rice cakes in a food processor or mini chopper until small crumbs form. Pour in a shallow bowl, add paprika and salt, and toss to combine.

2. Whisk egg and almond milk in a separate bowl. Dip tenderloins first into egg mixture and then into rice cake mixture, turning to coat.

3. Preheat oven to 375 degrees. Grease a baking sheet with non-stick spray and set aside.

4. Heat oil in a large, oven-safe skillet over medium heat, and brown tenderloins, about 5 minutes per side. Place on prepared baking sheet and bake until cooked through, about 8 minutes or until the internal temperature reaches 165 degrees.

5. While the turkey cooks, whisk together mustard, apricot spread, and lemon juice.

6. Serve tenderloins warm, with dipping sauce on side.

▶ SERVES 4

tip: If you do not have an oven-safe skillet, simply wrap plastic handle tightly with tinfoil.

2 rice cakes

1 teaspoon sweet paprika

½ teaspoon sea salt

1 large egg

2 teaspoons almond milk (NS substitute rice milk)

4 turkey tenderloins

1 tablespoon olive oil

dipping sauce:

2 teaspoons ground mustard

2 tablespoons no-sugar-added apricot spread (NS substitute plum jam)

1 teaspoon lemon juice

Type O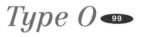

Shredded Turkey Bake

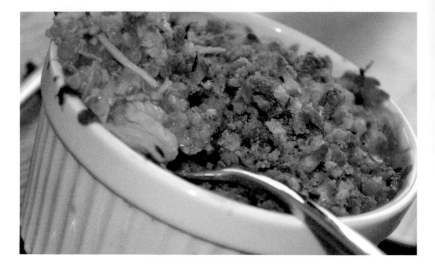

3 teaspoons olive oil, divided

1 cup diced carrots

1 cup diced onion

2 tablespoons plus 1 teaspoon fresh thyme, divided

2 cups carrot juice

1 cup Vegetable Stock*

Sea salt, to taste

1½ pounds turkey tenderloin

1 tablespoon arrowroot starch

2 tablespoons cold water

½ cup quinoa

1 cup quartered asparagus spears

1½ cups bread crumbs*

½ cup shredded mozzarella cheese (NS omit cheese or replace with shredded manchego cheese)

1. Heat 2 teaspoons olive oil in a Dutch oven over medium heat. Add carrots and onion and sauté for 5 minutes. Add 2 tablespoons thyme, carrot juice, stock, and salt, and stir just to combine. Add turkey tenderloin. Bring mixture to a boil, cover, reduce heat to a low simmer, and cook for 1½ hours.

2. Preheat oven to 375 degrees.

3. Remove turkey, place onto a cutting board and shred into bite-size pieces. Return to pot and increase heat to medium, letting carrot juice reduce by an inch. In a small bowl, dissolve arrowroot starch in water. Add to shredded turkey mixture, stir, and cook 10 minutes, to allow liquid to thicken. Add quinoa and cook an additional 12 minutes.

4. Mix bread crumbs with remaining 1 teaspoon olive oil, ⅛ teaspoon salt, and remaining 1 teaspoon fresh thyme. Toss with cheese.

5. Divide turkey mixture among 6 (7-oz.) ramekins, top with bread crumb mixture, and bake for 8 to 10 minutes or until turkey mixture is bubbling and topping is melted.

*See Vegetable Stock NS recipe (page 223). See Basic Gluten-Free Bread Crumbs NS recipe (page 224).

▶ SERVES 6

4 cups plus 1 tablespoon water

8 green tea bags

1 pound chicken breasts (4 pieces)

1 lemon, divided

½ teaspoon sea salt

1 cup fresh parsley

3 tablespoons olive oil

1 clove garlic

1. In a high-sided skillet, bring 4 cups of water to a boil and steep tea bags for 3 minutes. Slice half of lemon. Reduce skillet heat to medium and add chicken breasts, lemon slices, and sea salt. Cover and let cook 18 to 20 minutes, or until the internal temperature of chicken reaches 165 degrees.

2. Puree parsley, olive oil, garlic, remaining lemon juice, and remaining 1 tablespoon water in a food processor until very smooth.

3. Serve chicken warm, topped with parsley oil.

▶ SERVES 4

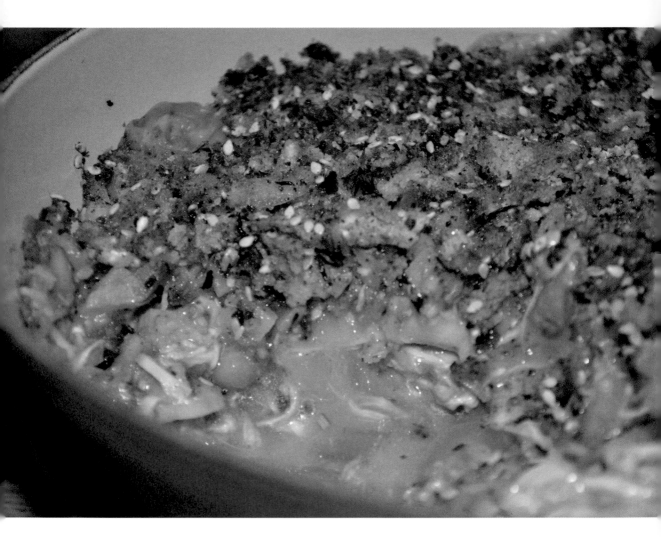

1. Preheat oven to 375 degrees.

2. Heat olive oil in a Dutch oven over medium heat and sauté onion, carrots, peas, and okra for 5 minutes. Sprinkle flour over vegetables, and add broth, stirring to prevent lumps. Add roasted chicken, saffron, and ground mustard, stirring to combine. Cover and let cook 15 minutes, stirring occasionally.

3. Heat olive oil in a large skillet over medium heat. Add Jerusalem artichokes, and sauté 3 to 4 minutes. Remove and toss with bread crumbs and sesame seeds. Drizzle with melted ghee.

4. Uncover chicken filling, and top with artichoke mixture. Place in the oven for 20 minutes, until pot pie is bubbling and topping is browned and crispy.

5. Serve warm.

*See Basic Gluten-Free Bread Crumbs NS recipe (page 224). See Chicken Stock recipe (page 221).

▶ **SERVES 8**

2 teaspoons olive oil

1 cup frozen pearl onions, thawed

1 cup diced baby carrots

1 cup sweet peas

1 cup chopped okra

2 tablespoons brown rice flour

3¼ cups chicken stock*

1½ pounds roasted chicken breast, shredded

¼ teaspoon saffron threads

½ teaspoon ground mustard

topping:

1 teaspoon olive oil

2 cups peeled and diced Jerusalem artichoke

½ cup bread crumbs*

2 tablespoons sesame seeds

2 teaspoons ghee, melted

featured ingredient

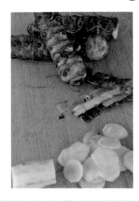

jerusalem artichokes

Crisp and crunchy, Jerusalem artichoke is a root vegetable with a beautiful, yellow flower resembling a sunflower. They have a slightly sweet, nutty flavor and can be used similar to potatoes or sliced thinly and fried. Neutral to most Type Os, Jerusalem artichokes are a fun, tasty new vegetable to get your hands on.

 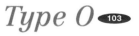

Broccolini-Stuffed Chicken

2 teaspoons ghee

1 bunch broccolini, roughly chopped

½ red onion, diced

Sea salt, to taste

¼ cup walnuts

⅓ cup crumbled feta cheese (NS omit cheese)

1 cup Vegetable Stock*, divided

1 pound skinless chicken breasts

1 tablespoon olive oil

1 tablespoon brown rice flour

1 tablespoon fresh oregano

1 tablespoon lemon juice

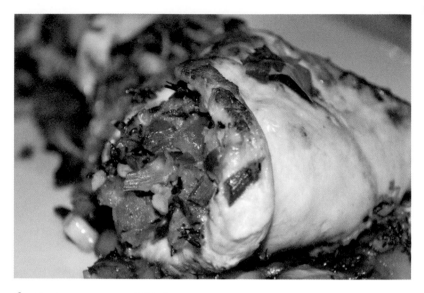

1. Preheat oven to 350 degrees.

2. Heat ghee in large skillet over medium heat. Sauté broccolini and onion until slightly tender, about 2 to 3 minutes. Season with salt, to taste.

3. Combine broccolini mixture, walnuts, cheese, and ¼ cup stock in a food processor, and pulse to combine. Filling should be thick and pasty but not too dry, similar in consistency to cookie dough. If mixture looks dry, add stock, 1 tablespoon at a time, to reach desired consistency. Set aside.

4. Butterfly the chicken by positioning the chicken breast with the tip facing you and the thickest part of the chicken breast facing your slicing hand. Put your hand on top of the chicken breast and insert the knife into the thickest part of the breast and carefully cut across the breast almost until you reach the opposite side, to create a pocket for the filling.

5. Divide broccolini stuffing among chicken breasts and secure breasts closed with toothpicks or cooking twine. Season outside of chicken breasts with sea salt.

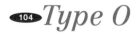

6. Heat olive oil in an oven-safe skillet over medium heat. Sear chicken breasts, about 2 minutes per side. Cover, place in the oven, and cook for 20 to 25 minutes, until juices run clear and the internal temperature of chicken reaches 165 degrees.

7. Remove from oven and transfer chicken breasts to a plate to rest. Place the skillet over medium heat and add flour. Gradually whisk in remaining stock, oregano, and lemon juice, bring to a simmer, and cook until thickened. Season with sea salt, to taste, and serve sauce over chicken.

*See Vegetable Stock NS recipe (page 223).

▶ SERVES 4

featured ingredient

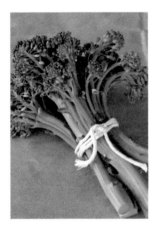

broccolini

Broccolini looks like an elongated and tender version of broccoli. Broccolini has a slightly more mild taste, however, and is much more palatable when sautéed, roasted, or grilled. If cooked simply, it pairs best with olive oil and garlic. Broccolini is often confused with rappini or broccoli rabe, which have a much more bitter taste and are less appealing to most people.

Beef Tips with Wild Mushrooms

NS

1 teaspoon paprika

½ teaspoon sea salt

½ teaspoon chili powder

1 teaspoon dried thyme

1½ pounds organic beef steak tips

3 teaspoons olive oil, divided

1 teaspoon ghee

1 cup diced onions

8 ounces cremini mushrooms, diced

2 cups diced maitake mushrooms

1 tablespoon fresh thyme

1. Combine paprika, sea salt, chili powder, and dried thyme in a small bowl. Sprinkle mixture evenly over beef, and rub in with your hands to evenly distribute.

2. Heat 2 teaspoons olive oil in a large sauté pan over medium heat, and brown beef, 2 to 3 minutes per side. Remove from pan and set aside.

3. In the same skillet, add remaining olive oil and ghee, and sauté onion, 3 to 4 minutes. Add mushrooms and fresh thyme, and sauté an additional 8 to 10 minutes. Return beef to the pan, and toss with mushrooms.

4. Serve warm.

▶ SERVES 4

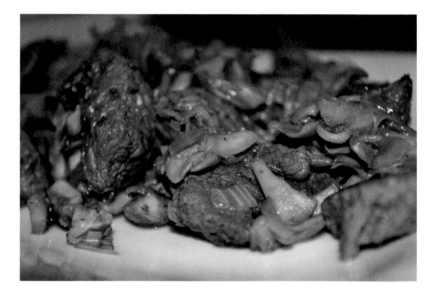

EAT RIGHT FOR YOUR TYPE PERSONALIZED COOKBOOK

Beef and Bean Chili

1. Heat olive oil in a large stockpot over medium heat. Add onion, garlic, and jalapenos, and sauté 4 to 5 minutes. Remove from pan and set aside.

2. In the same pot, add meat, and cook 5-6 minutes, breaking meat apart with a flat spatula as it browns. Once browned, add onion mixture back into the pot along with remaining ingredients. Cover and let simmer at least 45 minutes. Stir occasionally to prevent burning.

3. Serve warm.

▶ SERVES 4

2 teaspoons olive oil

2 cups chopped yellow onion

1 clove garlic, minced

2 jalapenos, finely diced

¾ pound lean ground beef

8 tomatoes, chopped

1 cup diced green bell pepper

1 cup diced red bell pepper

¼ teaspoon ground cinnamon (NS omit cinnamon)

1 teaspoon sea salt

2 teaspoons chili powder

1 teaspoon ground cumin

¼ cup tomato paste

1 can black beans, drained and rinsed

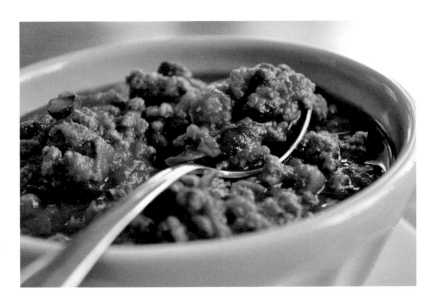

Type O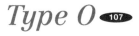

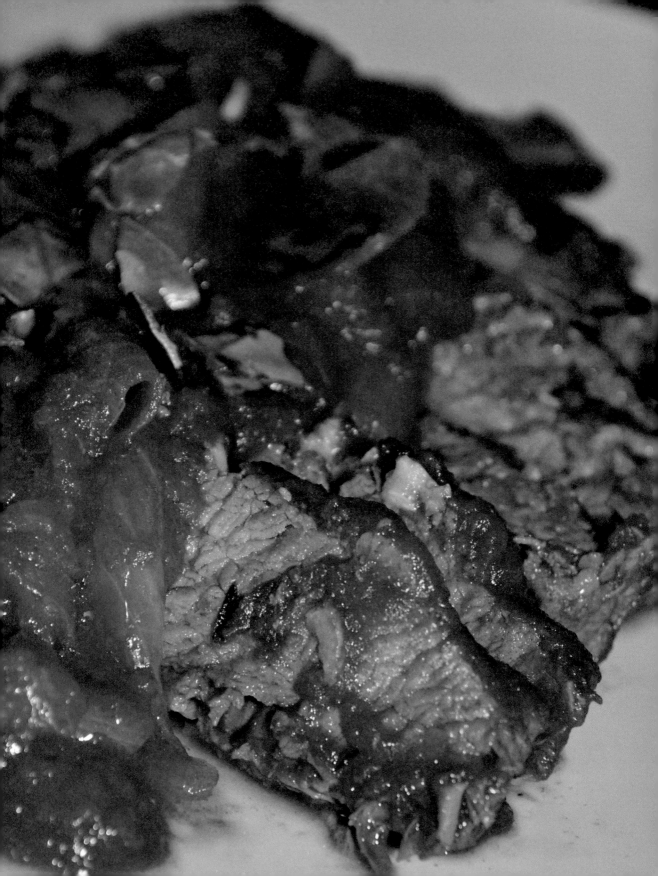

Braised Brisket

1. Preheat oven to 350 degrees.

2. Trim fat off brisket. Slice garlic into thin pieces. Using a paring knife, insert knife into brisket to create little pockets for the garlic, and insert garlic into the pockets. Sprinkle brisket with cumin, cinnamon, and sea salt.

3. In a large-bottomed skillet, heat olive oil over medium heat. Once hot, add brisket and brown on each side, 2-3 minutes. Place brisket into a roasting pan.

4. Add onions and carrots to the skillet, sauté 5 minutes, and add sea salt, to taste. Add red wine and tomato sauce, and stir to deglaze the bottom of pan.

5. Pour the mixture and fresh thyme around brisket. Add water to come about three-quarters the way up the sides of the brisket. Cover with parchment paper and tinfoil (tinfoil does not react well with the acidity in tomatoes, so the parchment paper should fully cover the beef), and bake for 3 hours.

6. Take brisket out of the oven, remove the meat, and let rest on a cutting board. Place the baking dish over medium heat on the stovetop to thicken the tomato sauce, about 5 minutes, stirring occasionally.

7. While the sauce thickens, slice brisket against the grain.

8. Serve warm, topped with tomato sauce.

▶ SERVES 6

3 pounds beef brisket

3 cloves garlic

1 teaspoon ground cumin

¼ teaspoon ground cinnamon (NS omit cinnamon, add less than ⅛ teaspoon cloves)

1 teaspoon sea salt

2 teaspoons olive oil

1 red onion, peeled and chopped

2 white onions, peeled and chopped

3 large carrots, peeled and chopped

½ cup red wine

2 cups stewed tomato sauce

4 large sprigs fresh thyme

¾ cup water

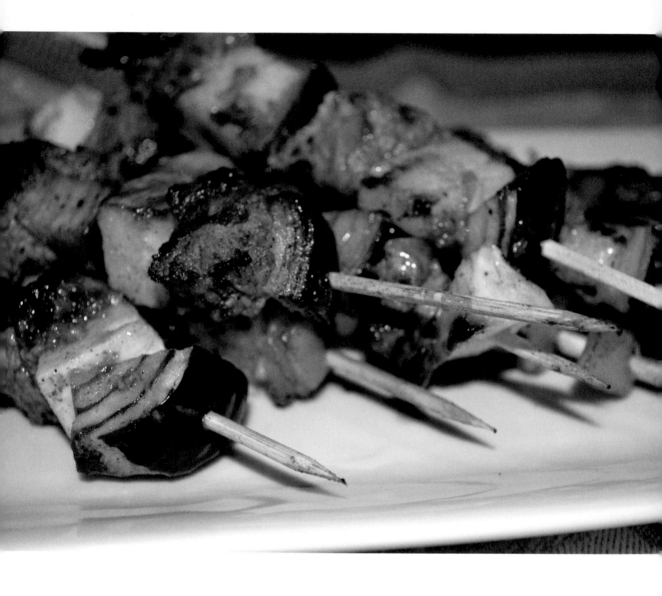

Tangy Pineapple and Beef Kabobs NS

1. Soak about 15 bamboo skewers in water for up to 1 hour before use to prevent burning.

2. Whisk together lemon juice, agave, olive oil, ginger, paprika, and garlic in a bowl.

3. Trim any excess fat off beef. Place in a glass storage dish with a sealable lid and pour two-thirds of the marinade over the beef, tossing to ensure all sides are coated. Cover and place in the refrigerator for 3 hours.

4. Preheat grill or grill pan to medium-high heat.

5. Alternate 2 pieces of steak, 2 pieces of pineapple, and 2 onion slices on each skewer. Brush pineapple and onion with marinade. Grill for 10 to 12 minutes, flipping halfway through cooking and brushing with any remaining marinade.

6. Serve warm.

▶ SERVES 4

marinade:

2 tablespoons fresh lemon juice

1 tablespoon agave

3 tablespoons olive oil

1 tablespoon minced fresh ginger

½ teaspoon sweet paprika

1 teaspoon garlic, minced

1 pound organic beef tips

4 cups pineapple pieces

1 red onion, cut into ½-inch dice

 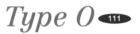

Sweet Potato Shepherd's Pie

2½ teaspoons olive oil, divided

3 cloves garlic, divided

Sea salt, to taste

2 medium sweet potatoes

1 tablespoon chopped fresh sage

1 tablespoon ghee or butter, divided

6 tablespoons almond milk (NS substitute rice milk)

1 pound ground beef

2 teaspoons paprika

2 tablespoons brown rice flour

1½ cups beef broth

2 cups pearl onions

1 cup peas

2 cups finely diced carrots

1 cup mozzarella cheese (NS omit cheese)

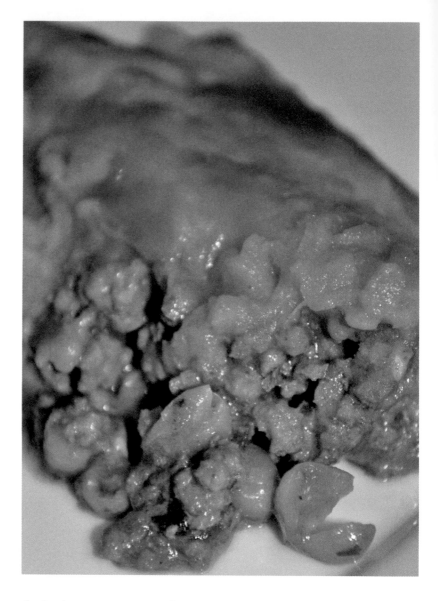

1. Preheat oven to 375 degrees.

2. Drizzle ½ teaspoon olive oil over 2 cloves of garlic, and season with sea salt. Wrap garlic in parchment paper and then tinfoil, and roast in the oven for 25 minutes. Remove from oven and set aside. Reduce oven temperature to 350 degrees.

3. Dice sweet potatoes into 2-inch pieces, place in a stockpot with enough water to cover. Bring to a boil and cook about 12 to 15 minutes, just until tender and easily pierced with a fork. Drain into a colander, and transfer back into the empty pot or a clean bowl. Using a hand mixer, beat sweet potatoes with roasted garlic, sage, ghee, and almond milk. Season with sea salt, to taste, and set aside.

4. Heat remaining olive oil in a large skillet over medium heat. Brown ground beef, 5-6 minutes, breaking into bits using a flat-ended spatula. Add paprika and flour, stirring to coat. Mince remaining clove of garlic, and add to the pot along with beef broth. Bring the mixture to a simmer, reduce heat to low, and cook for 5 minutes until mixture thickens.

5. Add onions, peas, and carrots and stir to combine. Pour into a 9" x 11" baking dish, and top with sweet potato mixture, spreading evenly across the top with an offset spatula. Sprinkle cheese over top and bake for 30 to 35 minutes, until pot pie is bubbling and cheese is melted and slightly browned.

6. Serve warm.

▶ SERVES 6

tip: Frozen pearl onions can be substituted in this recipe as a time-saver.

Sun-Dried Tomato Burgers on Millet Buns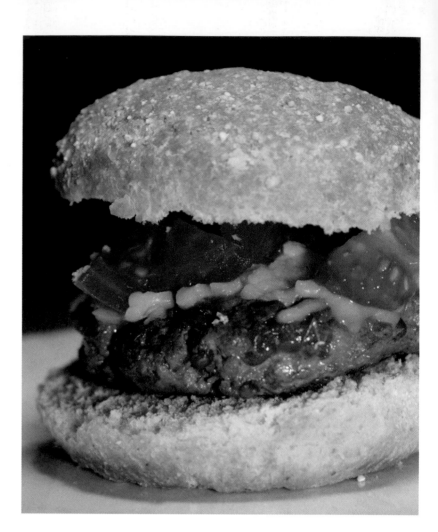

NS

2 tablespoons finely diced sun-dried tomato

1 pound lean ground beef

½ onion, grated

1 tablespoon fresh thyme

½ teaspoon sea salt

4 millet buns, toasted

1. Place sun-dried tomatoes in a small bowl and cover with very hot water. Let stand 10 minutes. Drain and pat dry.

2. Break ground beef into a large bowl. Add onion, sun-dried tomatoes, thyme, and salt. Using your hands, mix gently to combine, being careful not to overwork the meat. Form into 6 patties.

3. Heat a skillet or grill pan over medium heat, coat with non-stick olive oil spray. Cook 3 to 4 minutes per side.

4. Serve on toasted millet buns, with (allowable) cheese, diced tomatoes, caramelized onions, or Ketchup Substitute (page 218).

▶ SERVES 6

EAT RIGHT FOR YOUR TYPE PERSONALIZED COOKBOOK

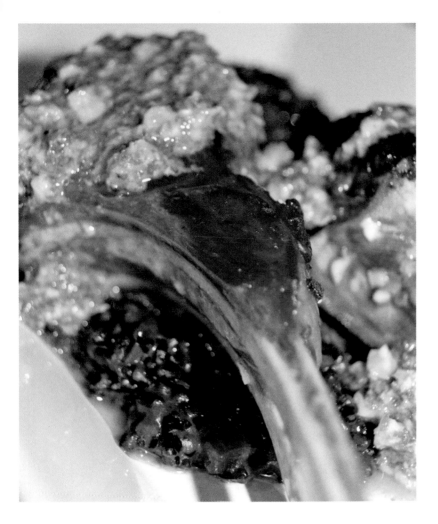

Grilled Lamb Chops with Mint Pesto 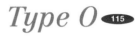 NS

1 pound lamb chops
Sea salt, to taste
½ cup olive oil, divided
3 cloves garlic, chopped

pesto:
½ cup fresh spinach
1 bunch fresh mint
1 teaspoon minced garlic
¼ cup extra virgin olive oil
½ teaspoon sea salt
Juice of 1 lemon
¼ cup raw walnuts

1. Season lamb with salt, place in a sealable glass container, and marinate with olive oil and garlic. Refrigerate at least 1 hour. Remove from fridge and let come to room temperature before using.

2. Place all pesto ingredients in a food processor, and pulse until smooth. Spoon into a small bowl and set aside.

3. Heat a grill pan over medium and brush with 1 tablespoon olive oil. Grill lamb 6 to 7 minutes on each side for medium doneness.

4. Top with pesto and serve with Forbidden Black Rice Risotto NS (page 157).

▶ SERVES 4

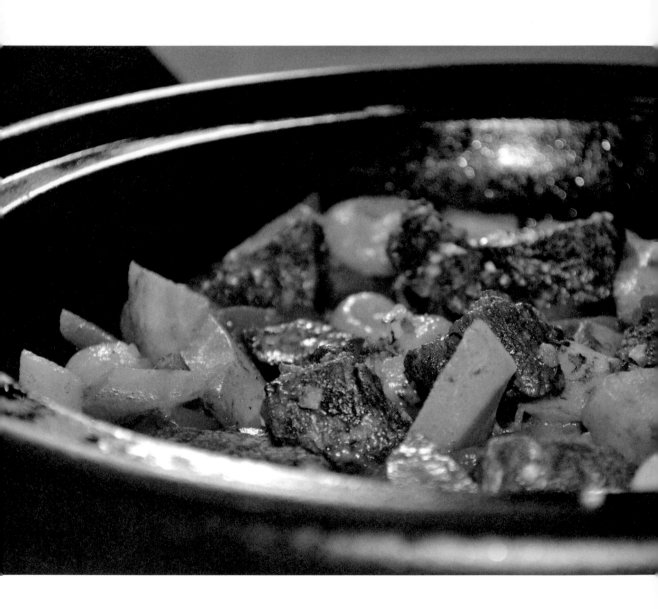

Moroccan Lamb Tagine

1. In a small bowl, combine garlic, ginger, cinnamon, cumin, and turmeric. Rub spices on lamb fillets. Heat tagine over medium-high heat, and brush with 1 teaspoon olive oil. Sear lamb just until browned on both sides, about 2 minutes. Remove lamb from tagine and set aside.

2. Add remaining 1 teaspoon olive oil, onions, carrots, and parsnips to the tagine, and cook 5 to 6 minutes.

3. Reduce heat to low. Place pieces of lamb back into the tagine on top of vegetables, and add stock and lemon juice. Cover and let cook for 1½ hours (and no peeking!).

4. After the time has elapsed, uncover and serve warm. Most of the liquid should be absorbed, and lamb and vegetables will be tender.

*See Vegetable Stock NS recipe (page 223).

▶ SERVES 4

2 teaspoons minced garlic

2 teaspoons minced ginger

¼ teaspoon ground cinnamon (NS omit cinnamon, add ⅛ teaspoon allspice)

¼ teaspoon ground cumin

½ teaspoon turmeric

8 ounces lamb fillet

2 teaspoons olive oil, divided

10 cipollini onions, peeled

1 cup chopped carrots

1 cup chopped parsnips

½ cup Vegetable Stock*

1 tablespoon lemon juice

tip: A tagine is a Moroccan cooking vessel that has a heavy, cast-iron or clay base and a domed, pyramid shaped top, which creates a slow cooking method that adds moisture to each dish. As an alternative, try a cast-iron skillet and cover with tented tinfoil, being sure to fully seal the top of the skillet.

 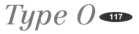

Slow-Cooker Venison NS

1 tablespoon olive oil plus 1 teaspoon, divided

1 cup chopped onion

1 cup chopped carrots

1 teaspoon sea salt

½ teaspoon paprika

2 teaspoons dried parsley

1 teaspoon garlic powder

12 ounces venison roast

1 cup beef broth

¼ cup red wine

1. Turn slow cooker to low setting.

2. Heat 2 teaspoons oil in a large skillet over medium heat. Sauté onion and carrots for 3 to 4 minutes. Remove vegetables from pan and place in slow cooker.

3. Combine salt, paprika, parsley, and garlic powder in a small bowl, stirring to combine. Sprinkle spices over roast and gently massage into all sides.

4. Add remaining olive oil (2 teaspoons) to skillet and increase temperature to medium to medium-high heat. Brown roast on all sides, cooking 1 to 2 minutes per side.

5. Remove roast from skillet and place in slow cooker. Pour beef broth and red wine into skillet to deglaze the pan and use a flat spatula to work up all the bits in the bottom of the pan. Pour broth and bits over roast in slow cooker. Cover and cook on low for 5 hours.

6. Serve warm with Brown Rice Salad NS (page 156).

▶ **SERVES 4**

Meat Loaf

1. Preheat oven to 375 degrees. Line a baking sheet with parchment paper and set aside.

2. Place all ingredients in a large bowl. Use your hands to mix just until incorporated, being careful not to overwork the meat.

3. Gather into a large ball, and place on prepared baking sheet. Form mixture into a log shape, and bake 45 minutes or until beef is no longer pink inside and juices run clear.

4. Serve warm.

*See Basic Gluten-Free Bread Crumbs NS recipe (page 224).

▶ SERVES 4

1 pound ground beef

1 cup diced onion

¼ cup finely diced carrot

¼ cup tomato paste

½ teaspoon mustard powder

1 clove garlic, minced

¼ teaspoon chili powder

1 teaspoon paprika

1 large egg, lightly beaten

1 cup bread crumbs*

 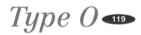

Red Quinoa–Mushroom Casserole with Fried Eggs NS

1 cup red quinoa

2 cups water

2 teaspoons ghee

1 cup diced maitake mushrooms

1½ cups diced okra

½ cup finely diced shallots

½ teaspoon mustard powder

½ teaspoon dry ginger

2 cloves garlic, minced

2 tablespoons fresh oregano, chopped

¾ cup finely diced pineapple

½ cup diced enoki mushrooms

1 cup Vegetable Stock*

5 eggs, divided

1 teaspoon olive oil

1. Preheat oven to 350 degrees. Grease a 9" x 11" baking dish with nonstick olive oil spray and set aside.

2. Bring quinoa and water to a boil, reduce to a simmer, and cook for 12 minutes. Remove from heat and fluff with a fork.

3. While quinoa cooks, melt ghee in a large skillet over medium heat. Add maitake mushrooms, okra, and shallots, and sauté 6 to 7 minutes.

4. In a small bowl, whisk mustard powder, ginger, garlic, oregano, pineapple, enoki mushrooms, stock, and 1 egg. Toss quinoa with mushroom mixture and place in prepared baking dish. Pour mixture evenly over casserole, and use a fork to make sure the liquid reaches all corners of the casserole.

5. Bake for 35 minutes, until casserole sets and becomes firm.

6. Just before removing casserole, heat olive oil in a large skillet over medium heat. Fry remaining eggs, and place on top of casserole.

7. Serve warm.

*See Vegetable Stock NS recipe (page 223).

▶ SERVES 6

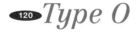

featured ingredient

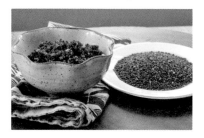

red quinoa

Red quinoa is almost identical in nutritional content to regular quinoa, and is a terrific source of fiber and protein, as it contains all nine essential amino acids. It also has a similar texture—light and fluffy with a slight crunch—to regular quinoa. The difference is that red quinoa has an earthier and less bitter taste. Use it in savory recipes, adding hearty vegetables, allowable cheeses, or beans.

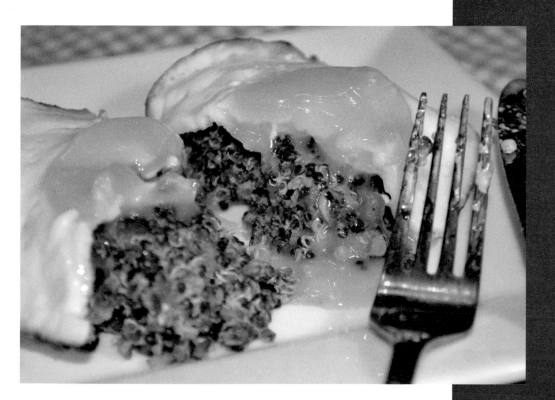

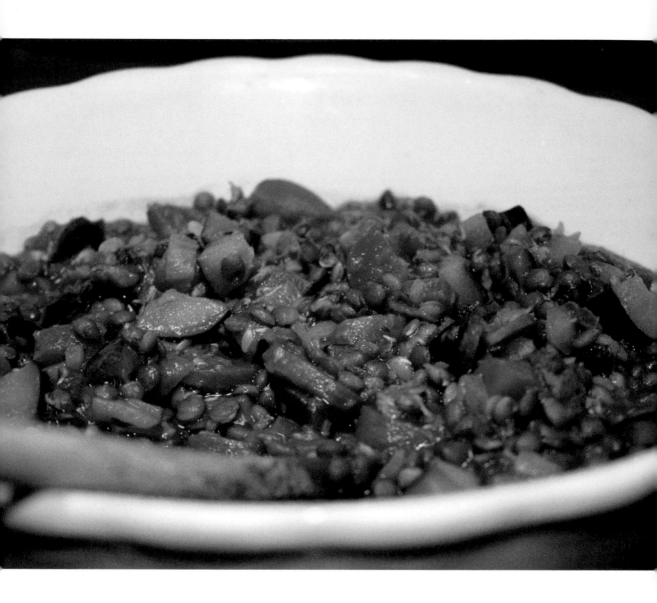

Sprouted Lentil Stew NS

1. Soak sprouted lentils in warm water for 25 minutes.

2. While the lentils soak, heat olive oil in a large Dutch oven over medium heat. Add onion, carrots, chilies, zucchini, and cumin, and sauté 6 to 7 minutes. Drain lentils and add to the Dutch oven with the other veggies and cook 1 minute, then add kombu and salt.

3. Add stock 1 cup at a time, stirring after each addition, and cook a total of 30 to 35 minutes.

4. Kombu will expand and then break apart into small pieces while cooking. (If this does not happen, remove, chop, and place back into the stew.)

5. Serve warm.

*See Vegetable Stock NS recipe (page 223).

▶ SERVES 4

1 cup sprouted lentils
1 tablespoon olive oil
1 cup diced onions
¾ cup diced carrots
1 tablespoon diced serrano chilies
2 zucchini, diced
½ teaspoon ground cumin
1 (4-inch) piece kombu
½ teaspoon sea salt
5 cups Vegetable Stock*

featured ingredient

sprouted lentils

Anytime you see the word *sprouted* in connection with a grain, legume, or seed it simply means that the food enzymes have been activated. This results in an increased nutrient content. Sprouted lentils can be found at most natural foods stores, and cook up much faster than lentils that have not been sprouted. They are a great addition to your "fast food" repertoire!

Spaghetti Squash with Goat Cheese and Walnuts

1 large spaghetti squash

1 tablespoon olive oil, divided

½ teaspoon large-grain sea salt

¼ cup very finely diced onion

3 ounces goat cheese (NS omit goat cheese)

1 cup toasted diced walnuts

1 cup finely diced parsley

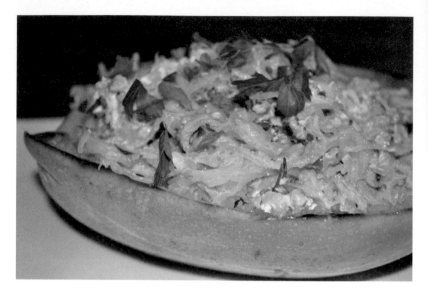

1. Preheat oven to 350 degrees.

2. Carefully halve squash from stem to base and scoop out seeds using a metal spoon. Brush 2 teaspoons olive oil and sprinkle sea salt over flesh of squash. Roast, cut side down, on a baking sheet for 35 to 40 minutes, until skin is browned, and flesh is easily pierced with a fork. Remove from oven and cool 5 minutes.

3. Heat remaining 1 teaspoon olive oil in a small skillet over medium heat. Sauté onion for 4 to 5 minutes, or until tender. Remove from heat, and add goat cheese, walnuts, and parsley.

4. Using a fork, scrape insides of squash from stem to base. Place strands of squash into a large bowl and toss with goat cheese mixture. (NS, once you have peeled squash into spaghetti strings, toss with 1 tablespoon olive oil, 1 tablespoon finely chopped basil, and remaining ingredients.)

5. Serve warm.

▶ SERVES 4

Soups and Sides

Thai Curry Soup NS ■ Carrot-Ginger Soup NS ■ Roasted Parsnip Soup ■ Melted Mozzarella–Onion Soup ■ Broccoli–Northern Bean Soup NS ■ Beef and Shredded Escarole Soup NS ■ Wild-Grain Soup with Sun-Dried Tomato Pesto NS ■ Tomato-Basil Soup NS ■ Sweet and Crunchy Kohlrabi Slaw NS ■ Sweet-and-Salty Brussels ■ Grilled Sesame-Ginger Bok Choy NS ■ South Indian–Curried Okra NS ■ Baked Beans NS ■ Spicy Collards NS ■ Garlic-Creamed Spinach ■ Roasted Escarole NS ■ Roasted Pumpkin with Fried Sage NS ■ Roasted Broccoli and Tomatoes NS ■ Sweet Potato Hash with Turkey Sausage ■ Autumn Roasted Roots NS ■ Rutabaga Smash ■ Whipped Sweet Potato Soufflé ■ Kohlrabi Gratin with Sage-Walnut Cream ■ Tomato and Broccoli Ragu NS ■ Creamy Rice Polenta ■ Brown Rice Salad NS ■ Forbidden Black Rice Risotto NS ■ Herbed Quinoa ■ Crisp-Tender Veggie Quinoa NS ■ Roasted Wakame and Fennel Salad NS ■ Mint and Cherry Tomato Tabbouleh NS

Many times when preparing dinner, we think about eating a protein, vegetable, and complex carbohydrate, and although having them all together in one pot like chili or lasagna is ideal, it doesn't always work out that way. Therefore, it is essential to have a collection of quick and delicious side or soup options to pair with your protein choice. A number of vegetable- or complex carbohydrate–based soups and sides to keep on hand can be found in this section.

Thai Curry Soup NS

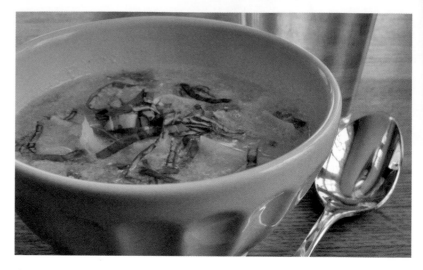

3 teaspoons olive oil

1 cup diced onion

1 teaspoon garlic, minced

1 tablespoon ginger, peeled and minced

⅛ teaspoon turmeric

½ teaspoon curry powder

1 jalapeno, cut into ¼-inch rounds

1 green bell pepper, diced into ½-inch cubes

2 small turnips, diced

Sea salt, to taste

1 stick lemongrass

4 cups water

cream sauce:

3 tablespoons chopped walnuts

2 tablespoons almond flour

1 teaspoon agave

3 tablespoons hot water or hot almond milk

1. Heat olive oil in a stockpot over medium heat. Sauté onion, garlic, and ginger for 3 to 4 minutes, until slightly tender and aromatic. Add turmeric, curry powder, jalapeno, bell pepper, and turnips, stir, and cook 5 minutes. Season with sea salt, to taste.

2. Trim ends of lemongrass and bruise stalk with the back of a knife to coax out the aroma and flavors. Pour water over vegetables, add lemongrass, cover, and simmer for at least 30 minutes.

3. While the soup simmers, place walnuts and almond flour in a food processor or mini chopper, and pulse until ingredients form a paste. Gradually drizzle in agave and hot water and puree until smooth and creamy.

4. Pour mixture into soup, and cook 5 minutes.

5. Remove lemongrass before serving. Serve warm.

▶ SERVES 6

featured ingredient

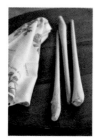

lemongrass

Lemongrass is a thick, woody stalk that needs to be bruised and chopped before use, to help bring out its flavor. For centuries, lemongrass has been thought to have healing properties. Lemongrass is most widely used in Asian cooking, and adds a fresh, citrus flavor to dishes.

EAT RIGHT FOR YOUR TYPE PERSONALIZED COOKBOOK

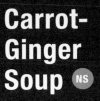

Carrot-Ginger Soup (NS)

1. Heat olive oil and ghee in a large stockpot over medium heat. Add onion, garlic, and carrots, and sauté 5 to 6 minutes, until vegetables become tender. Add remaining ingredients and bring to a boil, cover, reduce to a simmer, and cook at least 30 minutes, or until carrots are fork-tender.

2. Puree soup with an immersion blender or in batches in standing blender until smooth. Add water until consistency is the thickness of cake batter.

3. Serve warm.

▶ SERVES 6

1 teaspoon olive oil

2 teaspoons ghee

1 cup chopped onion

1 clove garlic

2 pounds carrots, peeled and diced

1 (3-inch) piece (or about ¼ cup) ginger, peeled and grated

½ teaspoon sea salt

1 tablespoon lemon zest

4 cups water

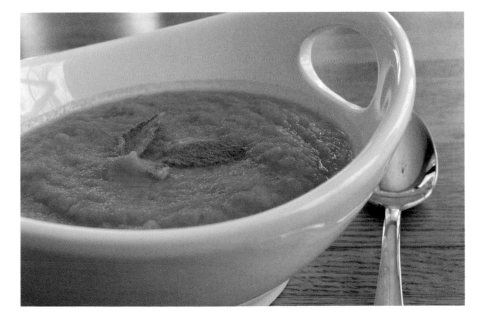

 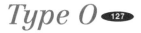

Roasted Parsnip Soup

4 cups diced parsnips

4 cups diced cauliflower

2 cloves garlic, peeled

2 tablespoons olive oil, divided

Sea salt, to taste

2 cups finely sliced sweet onion

2 finely diced Granny Smith apples

1½ cups soy or almond milk (NS substitute rice milk)

1 cup water

⅛ teaspoon nutmeg

¼ cup chopped fresh sage

1. Preheat oven to 375 degrees.

2. Place parsnips, cauliflower, and garlic on a sheet pan, drizzle with 1 tablespoon olive oil and sprinkle with sea salt. Toss to coat.

3. Roast vegetables in the oven for 35 to 40 minutes, or until tender and golden brown around the edges.

4. About 15 minutes before the vegetables are finished cooking in the oven, heat remaining 1 tablespoon olive oil in a large stockpot to medium heat. Sauté onion for 8 to 10 minutes, then add apples and sauté an additional 3 to 4 minutes.

5. Add roasted vegetables and remaining ingredients to pot. Bring the soup to a gentle boil, reduce heat, and simmer for 20 minutes. Blend with an immersion blender or puree in batches in a standing blender. Season with additional sea salt, to taste.

6. Serve warm.

▶ SERVES 6

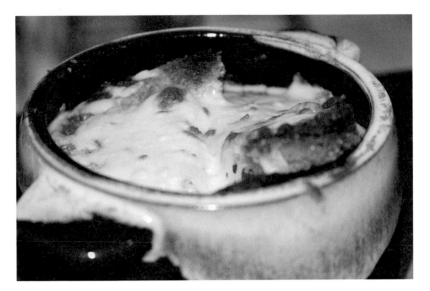

Melted Mozzarella– Onion Soup

1. Peel onions, slice in half and then slice in thin, half-moon shapes.

2. Heat olive oil and ghee in a large-bottomed stockpot over medium heat, add onions, and cook for 12 minutes, to caramelize. Season with sea salt, reduce temperature to medium-low, and cook 20 minutes, until onions are a rich, caramel color.

3. Add wine to pan, and cook 30 seconds. Add thyme, sage, bay leaves, salt, and broth. Simmer for 30 minutes. Remove bay leaves after cooking.

4. Preheat broiler. Divide soup among 4 (7-oz.) high-sided, oven-safe bowls or ramekins. Top each ramekin with 1 slice of toast, then sprinkle with cheese to create a cheesy bread lid for the soup.

5. Broil for 2 minutes or until the cheese begins to bubble and brown slightly. Keep a close eye on the broiler as the bread and cheese can burn quickly.

6. Serve warm.

▶ SERVES 4

5 large white onions

1 tablespoon olive oil

½ tablespoon ghee or butter

Sea salt, to taste

½ cup red wine

4 sprigs thyme

2 sprigs sage

2 bay leaves

3 cups beef broth

4 slices brown rice/millet bread.

1 cup grated mozzarella cheese (NS substitute manchego cheese)

Broccoli–Northern Bean Soup NS

1 tablespoon olive oil, divided

1 cup diced white onion

2 heads broccoli

1 clove garlic, minced

1 (15-oz.) can northern beans, drained and rinsed

2 cups Vegetable Stock*

4 sprigs fresh thyme

Sea salt, to taste

¼ cup pine nuts

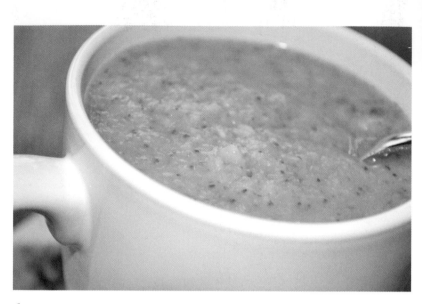

1. Heat 2 teaspoons olive oil in a large stockpot over medium heat, and sauté onion, 5 to 6 minutes.

2. Trim woody stems off broccoli and discard. Rough chop broccoli and remaining stems. Add to the onions along with garlic, beans, stock, and thyme. Bring to a boil, reduce heat, and simmer for 15 minutes, until vegetables are tender and easily pierced with a fork but not falling apart.

3. Puree soup using an immersion blender, or in batches using a stand blender. Soup should be thick and creamy, but easily run off a spoon. Add water or additional stock if you prefer a thinner consistency. Season with sea salt, to taste.

4. Heat remaining 1 teaspoon olive oil in a small skillet over medium heat. Toast pine nuts for 2 to 3 minutes, or until golden brown.

5. Serve soup hot, topped with toasted pine nuts.

*See Vegetable Stock NS recipe (page 223).

▶ SERVES 6

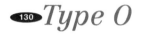

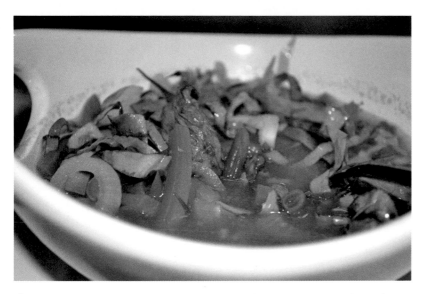

Beef and Shredded Escarole Soup NS

1. Heat 1 teaspoon olive oil in a Dutch oven over medium heat. Sauté ginger and garlic for 1 minute, stirring continuously to prevent burning.

2. Trim excess fat from beef and slice as thin as possible. Add remaining 1 teaspoon olive oil to skillet and add beef, cooking until browned, 3 to 4 minutes.

3. Add broth, water, onions, carrots, and bay leaf. Cook 20 minutes.

4. Remove bay leaf, add beans to soup, and cook 10 minutes. Spoon into bowls, and top each with ½ cup escarole.

▶ SERVES 4

2 teaspoons olive oil, divided

1 (1-inch) piece fresh ginger, peeled and minced

1 clove garlic, minced

¾ pound lean beef

Sea salt, to taste

2 cups organic beef broth

3 cups water

1 cup pearl onions

1 cup carrots, cut into matchsticks

1 bay leaf

2 cups haricot vert

2 cups shredded escarole

 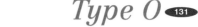

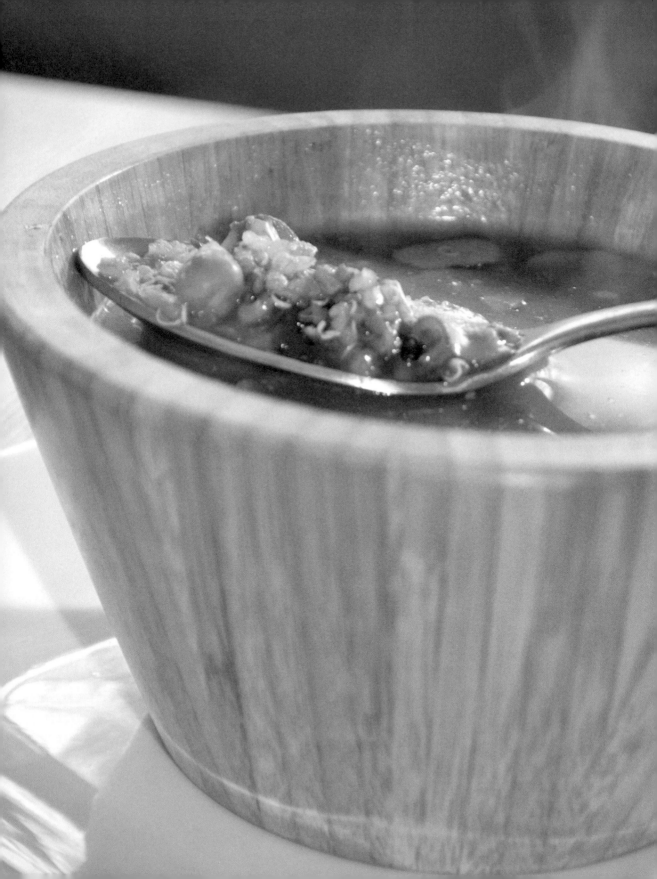

Wild-Grain Soup with Sun-Dried Tomato Pesto NS

1. Cook wild rice according to package instructions. Transfer to a bowl and set aside.

2. Melt ghee in a medium stockpot over medium heat, add garlic and mushrooms, and sauté 3 to 4 minutes. Add stock and water, bring to boil, reduce heat to a simmer, and cook 5 minutes.

3. While the soup simmers, combine sun-dried tomatoes, basil, garlic, olive oil, lemon juice, walnuts, water, and tomato paste in a food processor, and pulse to combine. Season with sea salt, to taste, and set aside.

4. Add quinoa and sea salt, to taste, to soup, and simmer an additional 10 minutes, until quinoa is tender.

5. Add snow peas and cooked rice, cook 3 minutes. Divide soup evenly among bowls and serve warm with a dollop of pesto.

*See Vegetable Stock NS recipe (page 223).

▶ SERVES 6

½ cup wild brown rice

2 teaspoons ghee

1 clove garlic

8 ounces cremini mushrooms

4 cups Vegetable Stock*

3 cups water

pesto:

½ cup sun-dried tomatoes

½ cup fresh basil

1 clove garlic

2 tablespoons olive oil

2 tablespoons lemon juice

¼ cup raw walnuts

3 tablespoons water

1 tablespoon tomato paste

Sea salt, to taste

¼ cup quinoa

¾ cup snow peas

Type O 133

Tomato-Basil Soup NS

1 teaspoon ghee

1 teaspoon extra virgin olive oil

1 white onion, chopped

1 teaspoon garlic, minced

8 vine-ripened tomatoes, diced

Sea salt, to taste

½ cup chopped fresh basil, divided

1. Melt ghee and olive oil in a Dutch oven over medium heat. Add onion and cook 4 to 5 minutes stirring frequently. Add garlic and stir an additional 30 seconds. Add tomatoes, and sea salt, to taste.

2. Simmer for 30 minutes. Stir in ¼ cup basil, then blend with an immersion blender or puree in batches in a standing blender.

3. Top with remaining basil and serve warm.

▶ **SERVES 4**

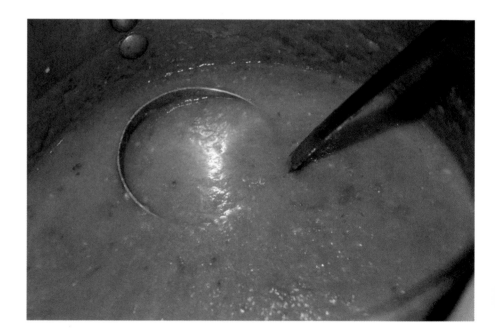

1. Whisk lemon juice, olive oil, mustard, honey, and sea salt in a large bowl and set aside.

2. Cut tough bottoms off the kohlrabi as well as stems coming off the top, and peel outer layer. Place grated broccoli and kohlrabi in bowl with dressing.

3. Add raisins and parsley, and toss to combine. Serve chilled.

▶ SERVES 4

tip: Reserve broccoli and kohlrabi tops, and sauté in a skillet with 1 tablespoon olive oil over medium heat for 5 to 8 minutes or until crisp-tender.

3 tablespoons lemon juice

3 tablespoons olive oil

2 teaspoons ground mustard

1 teaspoon honey or agave

Sea salt, to taste

2 cups grated kohlrabi (about 3 bulbs)

2 cups grated broccoli stems (about 2 bunches)

½ cup golden raisins

¼ cup chopped parsley

 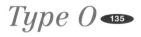

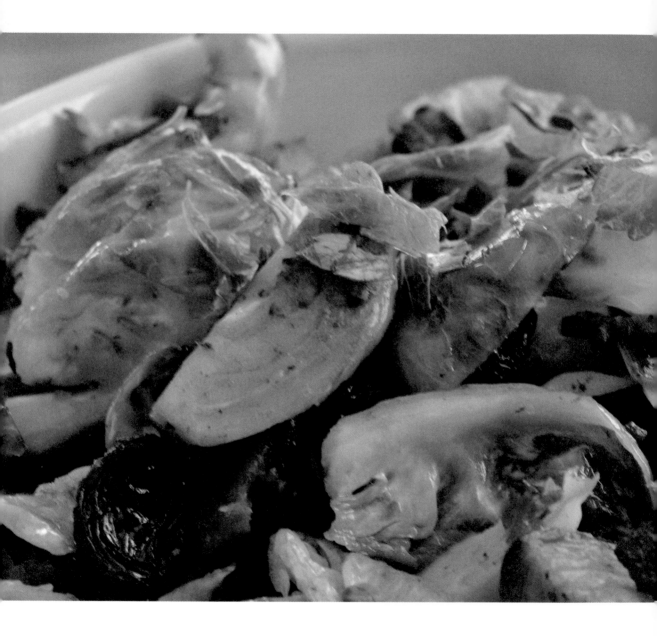

1 teaspoon ghee

2 teaspoons olive oil

2 tablespoons finely diced shallots

4 strips turkey bacon, diced

4 cups quartered Brussels sprouts

¼ cup golden raisins

½ cup Vegetable Stock*

1 tablespoon chopped parsley, for garnish

1. Melt ghee and olive oil in a large skillet over medium heat. Sauté shallots and turkey bacon until bacon is crispy, about 4 to 5 minutes.

2. Add Brussels sprouts and cook for 15 minutes, stirring occasionally to prevent burning.

3. Add raisins and stock and cook an additional 3 minutes, until raisins are tender and the broth can help deglaze the bottom of the pan.

4. Sprouts are done when they can be pierced with a fork but still give moderate resistance. Be careful to avoid overcooking, as they can become mushy and lose a lot of flavor.

5. Garnish with parsley and serve warm.

*See Vegetable Stock NS recipe (page 223).

▶ SERVES 4

Grilled Sesame-Ginger Bok Choy (NS)

2 teaspoons olive oil

1 teaspoon sesame oil

1 tablespoon fresh grated ginger

1 large bunch bok choy

Sea salt, to taste

1 teaspoon sesame seeds

1. In a small bowl, whisk olive oil, sesame oil, and ginger, and set aside.

2. Pull the leaves off the base of the bok choy and slice off the very bottom of the stem to remove any tough pieces. Wash leaves individually and let them dry completely on a kitchen towel.

3. Preheat grill pan over medium heat.

4. Brush individual bok choy leaves with sesame mixture.

5. Grill leaves for about 1 minute per side, until bok choy is wilted and stems and leaves are slightly browned. Sprinkle with sesame seeds and serve warm.

▶ SERVES 4

tip: When purchasing bok choy, look for stalks that are bright white in color with dark-green leaves. Avoid spotted stems and wilted-looking leaves.

EAT RIGHT FOR YOUR TYPE PERSONALIZED COOKBOOK

South Indian–Curried Okra NS

1 tablespoon olive oil

½ teaspoon mustard seeds

½ teaspoon ground cumin

2 teaspoons blanched almonds

¾ cup finely diced onion

3 cups diced okra

3 heirloom tomatoes, diced

½ teaspoon turmeric

½ teaspoon sea salt

1 teaspoon red chili powder

1. Heat olive oil in a Dutch oven over medium heat. Add mustard seeds, cumin, and almonds, and cook 30 seconds, stirring continuously to prevent burning. Add onion, and cook 5 minutes.

2. Add okra, and cook an additional 15 minutes, stirring occasionally.

3. Add tomatoes, turmeric, sea salt, and chili powder, and cook 5 to 8 minutes, until tomatoes break down into a sauce and okra is fork-tender.

4. Serve warm.

▶ SERVES 6

Baked Beans NS

2 teaspoons olive oil

1 cup diced yellow onion

1 clove garlic, minced

1 teaspoon dry mustard

1 teaspoon molasses

1 teaspoon salt

1 teaspoon paprika

½ teaspoon chili powder

2 cans adzuki beans, drained and rinsed

3 tablespoons tomato paste

⅓ cup Vegetable Stock*

1. Preheat oven to 375 degrees.

2. Heat olive oil in a Dutch oven over medium heat, and add olive oil. Sauté onion and garlic for 5 to 7 minutes, until translucent and tender. Add mustard, molasses, salt, paprika, and chili powder, and cook 1 additional minute.

3. Add adzuki beans, tomato paste, and stock, and stir to combine.

4. Cover and bake for 25 minutes, until mixture is thick and hot throughout.

5. Serve warm.

*See Vegetable Stock NS recipe (page 223).

▶ SERVES 6

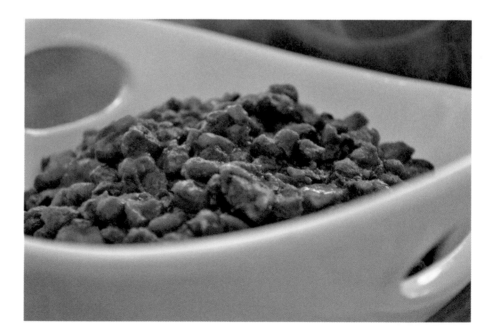

EAT RIGHT FOR YOUR TYPE PERSONALIZED COOKBOOK

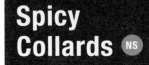
1. Melt olive oil and ghee in a large skillet over medium heat. Add shallots and bacon, and sauté until bacon is crispy, about 4 to 5 minutes.

2. Season with chili powder, and add collard greens. Cook 10 to 12 minutes, until collards are tender and slightly wilted.

3. Add black-eyed peas, and cook an additional 3 to 4 minutes, until warmed through.

4. Season with sea salt, to taste, and serve warm.

▶ SERVES 4

2 teaspoons olive oil

1 teaspoon ghee

½ cup diced shallots

4 slices turkey bacon, finely diced

½ teaspoon chipotle chili powder

1 bunch collard greens

1 (15-oz.) can black-eyed peas, drained and rinsed

Sea salt, to taste

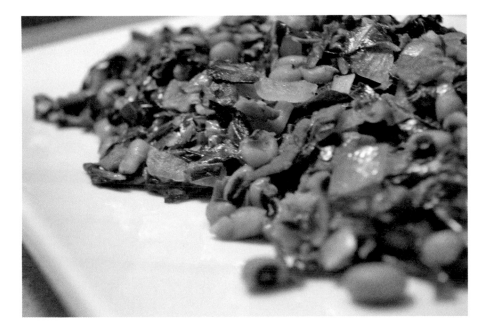

 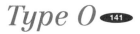

Garlic-Creamed Spinach

2 cups red, yellow, or red baby heirloom tomatoes or cherry tomatoes

2 teaspoons olive oil

Sea salt, to taste

1 tablespoon ghee

2 cloves garlic, minced

1 cup finely diced white onion

3 tablespoons brown rice flour

½ cup almond milk (NS substitute rice milk)

¾ cup Vegetable Stock*

10 cups roughly chopped baby spinach

1. Preheat oven to 400 degrees.

2. Halve tomatoes and toss with olive oil and sea salt. Spread in a single layer on a baking sheet and bake on the top rack of oven for 25 minutes.

3. While the tomatoes roast, melt ghee in a Dutch oven over medium heat, and sauté garlic and onion for 5 to 6 minutes Add brown rice flour and stir for 1 minute. Slowly add milk and stock, whisking continuously to avoid lumps. Continue whisking until mixture becomes the consistency of yogurt, about 5 minutes. Add spinach, approximately 2 cups at a time, allowing each batch to cook down slightly to make room for the next batch.

4. Add tomatoes to spinach mixture and serve warm.

*See Vegetable Stock NS recipe (page 223).

▶ SERVES 4

Roasted Escarole (NS)

1. Preheat oven to 375 degrees.

2. Trim woody stems off the bottom of escarole and roughly chop. Toss with olive oil and season with sea salt.

3. Spread escarole on 2 baking sheets and bake for 10 to 12 minutes, tossing after 5 minutes to help the escarole become crispy. Escarole should be dark green, wilted, and have crispy, slightly browned edges.

4. Serve immediately.

▶ SERVES 4

2 heads escarole, washed and dried

2 teaspoons olive oil

¼ teaspoon large-grain sea salt

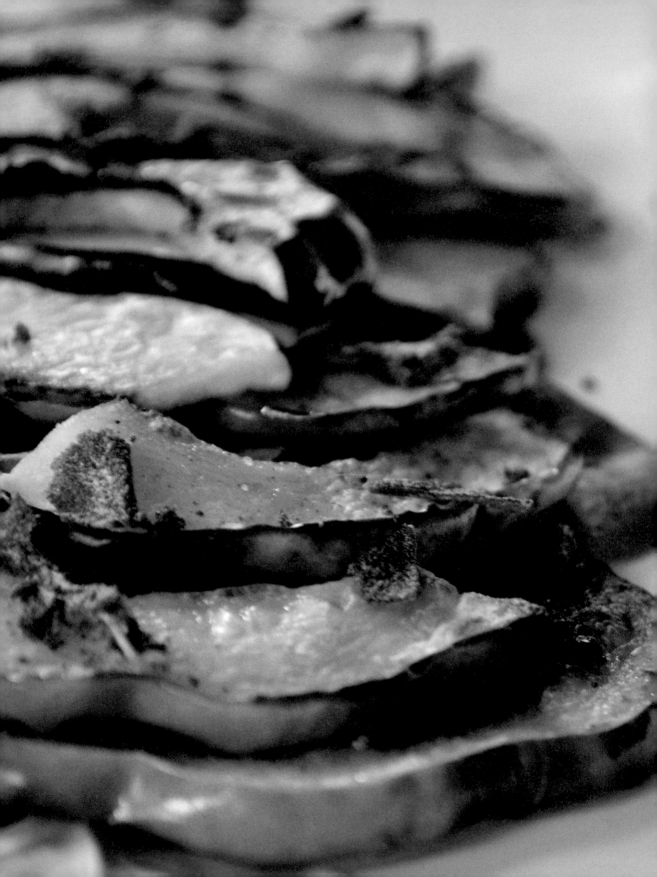

Roasted Pumpkin with Fried Sage (NS)

1. Preheat oven to 400 degrees.

2. Very carefully cut the top off the pumpkin and then slice in half vertically. Using a large metal spoon, remove all seeds and membranes from each half. Turn pumpkin cut side down on the cutting board for stability and slice into ½-inch sections. Repeat with remaining pumpkin half. Place pumpkin in a single layer on a baking sheet, drizzle with 2 teaspoons olive oil, a dash of sea salt, and nutmeg.

3. Roast for 45 to 50 minutes or until fork-tender.

4. Heat remaining 1 tablespoon olive oil in a small skillet over medium heat. Inspect sage leaves, and dry thoroughly if any water clings to them. (Wetness will splatter the hot oil.) Add sage and fry until crispy, 30 seconds. Remove with a slotted spoon to a paper towel, crumble, and set aside.

5. Garnish pumpkin with sage, and serve immediately.

▶ SERVES 4

1 (4-lb.) sugar pumpkin

⅛ teaspoon nutmeg

1 tablespoon plus 2 teaspoons olive oil, divided

2 tablespoons fresh sage

Sea salt, to taste

tip: When choosing a pumpkin to roast, opt for a smaller sugar pumpkin because it will have a sweeter flavor. Make sure there are no bruises or weak spots in the flesh and it feels firm. Using younger pumpkins is preferable as well because as pumpkins get older, their skin becomes tough and more difficult to work with.

Roasted Broccoli and Tomatoes NS

1 head broccoli

2 pints cherry tomatoes

2 teaspoons olive oil

Sea salt, to taste

1 clove garlic

1 tablespoon finely chopped basil, for garnish

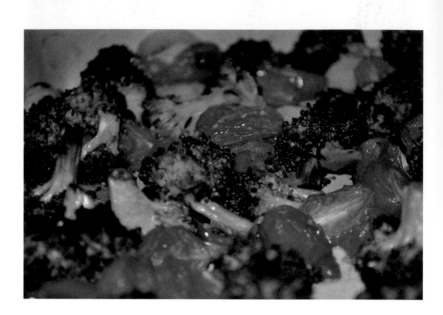

1. Preheat oven to 375 degrees.

2. Dice broccoli into bite-size pieces, and toss with tomatoes, olive oil, and sea salt. Place on a sheet pan or baking dish, and roast for 25 minutes.

3. Remove from the oven, and add garlic. Toss to evenly coat. Place back in the oven, and roast an additional 5 to 10 minutes, until tomatoes collapse and are blistered, and broccoli has slightly crispy, brown edges.

4. Remove from oven and garnish with basil.

▶ SERVES 4

tip: Eating tomato and broccoli together in the same dish increases the body's ability to absorb the nutrients that each vegetable supplies.

Sweet Potato Hash with Turkey Sausage

1. Slice sweet potatoes into about 2"x ¼" matchsticks. Place sweet potatoes in a large pot with enough cold water to cover, and bring to a boil. As soon as the water boils, drain, spread sweet potatoes out on a baking sheet lined with a clean kitchen towel, and let dry.

2. Melt ghee in a skillet over medium heat, and sauté onion and bell pepper for 3 to 4 minutes, until tender. Season with sea salt to taste. Remove turkey sausages from casing and add to onions. Break apart sausage with a flat-ended spatula and cook until browned, 4-5 minutes.

3. Remove mixture from pan, and set aside. Drizzle olive oil into skillet, add sweet potatoes, and let cook, undisturbed, for 2 minutes to brown potatoes. Flip and cook, undisturbed, 2 to 3 minutes to brown opposite side. Add sausage mixture, cinnamon, and maple syrup to the pan, and stir gently, just to combine.

4. Serve hot.

▶ SERVES 6

6 cups sliced sweet potatoes

2 teaspoons ghee

1 cup diced onion

1 cup diced green bell pepper

2 links turkey sausage

2 teaspoons olive oil

Sea salt, to taste

½ teaspoon ground cinnamon (NS omit cinnamon)

1 tablespoon maple syrup (NS substitute 1 teaspoon molasses and 2 teaspoons agave)

 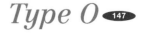

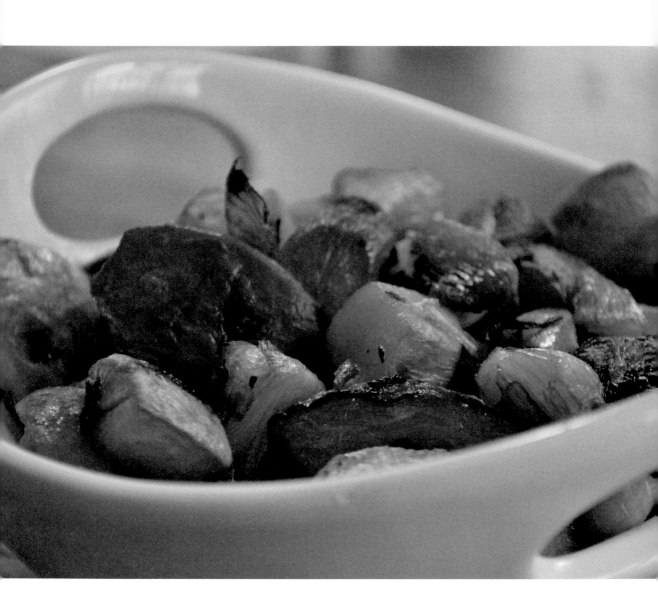

Autumn Roasted Roots (NS)

1. Preheat oven to 400 degrees.

2. Peel celery root, turnip, pumpkin, and carrots, and dice into 2-inch pieces.

3. Toss vegetables, shallots, olive oil, sea salt, and sage in a large bowl until combined.

4. Pour onto a baking sheet, and bake for 55 to 60 minutes, until vegetables are browned and crispy on the edges and soft inside.

5. Serve warm.

▶ SERVES 4

1 celery root
1 turnip
1 (3-lb.) sugar pumpkin
2 carrots
4 shallots, diced
1 tablespoon olive oil
1 teaspoon sea salt
2 tablespoons fresh, chopped sage

featured ingredient

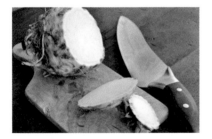

celery root

Otherwise known as celeriac, celery root is just that: the root of a type of celery. It has a deliciously fresh flavor that is a cross between celery and parsley, but works terrifically as a base for soups with onions and carrots, eaten raw, or roasted (as featured here). A *Neutral* for all blood types, celery root adds a diversity of flavor to your palate.

 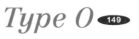

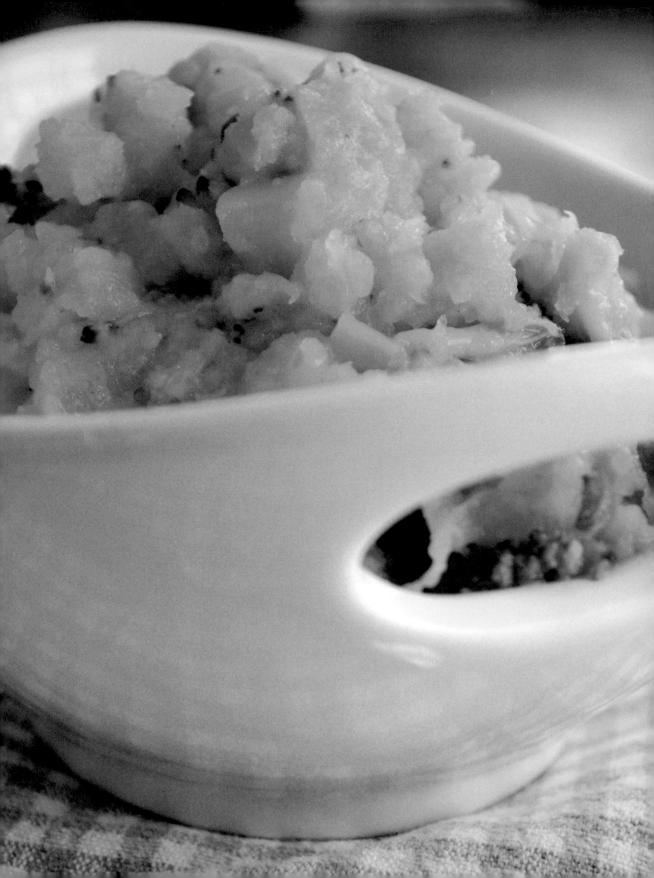

Rutabaga Smash

1. Peel rutabaga and dice into bite-size pieces. Place rutabaga in a pot with enough cold, salted water to cover, and bring to a boil. Cover, reduce heat, and simmer for 35 minutes, or until rutabaga is fork-tender.

2. While the rutabaga simmers, trim stems off broccoli and dice into bite-size pieces and coat with olive oil. Bring a pot of salted water to a boil, and steam for 5 to 6 minutes, until bright green and slightly tender. Drain and set aside.

3. When the rutabaga is finished cooking, drain, place the rutabaga back into the pot, and return to stove. Using a potato masher or fork, mash rutabaga, and add parsley, milk, garlic, ghee, and salt, to taste. Cook 3 to 4 minutes until ghee melts and flavors incorporate.

4. Fold broccoli in rutabaga mash.

5. Serve warm.

▶ SERVES 4

2 rutabaga roots
1 head broccoli
½ teaspoon olive oil
¼ cup roughly chopped parsley
¼ cup almond milk
2 cloves garlic, peeled
2 teaspoons ghee or butter
Sea salt, to taste

Whipped Sweet Potato Soufflé

1½ cups almond milk (NS substitute rice milk)

2 sprigs plus 1 tablespoon fresh sage, divided

3 egg yolks

¼ cup brown rice flour

1 tablespoon maple syrup

1 cup sweet potato, baked

1 tablespoon ghee or butter plus more for greasing

¼ teaspoon ground cinnamon (NS substitute ⅛ teaspoon nutmeg)

1 teaspoon sea salt

6 egg whites

tip: Egg whites cannot be beaten in a bowl that holds fat, such as plastic, so use a glass or copper one instead. Water inside the bowl will also prohibit egg whites from stiffening, so be sure to carefully wipe down the inside of the bowl before using.

1. Preheat oven to 350 degrees. Grease bottoms and sides of 8 (4-oz.) ramekins with ghee, and set aside.

2. In a small saucepan, combine milk with 2 sprigs of sage, and cook over low heat for 10 to 12 minutes. Remove sage after cooking.

3. Whisk together egg yolks, brown rice flour, and maple syrup in a small bowl. When milk is ready, temper egg yolks by very slowly pouring about ½ cup milk into the egg mixture, stirring continuously. Pour the tempered eggs back into the saucepan with the remaining milk, and stir over medium heat until thickened, 2 to 3 minutes.

4. Finely chop remaining 1 tablespoon sage.

5. Beat baked sweet potato with ghee, chopped sage, cinnamon, and salt in a medium bowl. When milk mixture has thickened, remove from heat and whisk in whipped sweet potato until smooth. Cool mixture completely.

6. In a dry, glass, stainless steel, or copper bowl, beat egg whites until they form stiff peaks. Fold egg whites into cooled sweet potato mixture, one-third at a time. Divide sweet potato mixture evenly among prepared ramekins, filling each three-quarters full.

7. Place ramekins in a high-sided baking dish, and place in the oven with the oven rack extended out of the oven. Pour hot water into the bottom of the baking dish to reach 1 inch. Bake soufflés for 55 to 60 minutes or until firm.

8. Serve immediately.

▶ SERVES 6

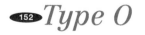 *Type O*

EAT RIGHT FOR YOUR TYPE PERSONALIZED COOKBOOK

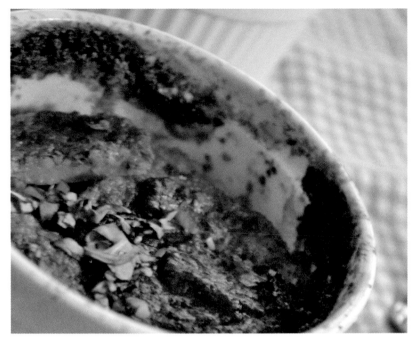

Kohlrabi Gratin with Sage-Walnut Cream

2 bulbs kohlrabi

½ cup almond milk (NS substitute rice milk)

⅛ teaspoon ground cloves

2 tablespoons fresh sage

¼ cup water

½ cup chopped walnuts

Sea salt, to taste

1 cup mozzarella cheese (NS substitute manchego cheese)

1. Preheat oven to 375 degrees.

2. Peel kohlrabi and slice off woody bottoms. Place in a pot with enough water to cover by 1 inch, bring to a boil, and cook for 6 to 7 minutes. Drain, slice kohlrabi into ¼-inch-thick rounds, and set aside.

3. In a small saucepan, combine almond milk, cloves, sage, and water, and bring to a boil. Reduce heat, and simmer until ready to use.

4. Pulse walnuts in a food processor until finely chopped. With the processor running, drizzle in half of the hot milk mixture and puree until walnut cream is the thickness of buttermilk. Add sea salt, to taste.

5. Spoon a small amount of walnut cream in the bottom of 2 (12-oz.) ramekins. Layer kohlrabi with walnut cream and shredded cheese, and repeat, until ramekins are filled to the top, finishing with cream and cheese. Pour remaining milk mixture evenly over ramekins, and bake for 30 to 35 minutes, until gratin is tender and bubbling, and the cheese is slightly browned and melted.

6. Serve warm.

▶ SERVES 4

 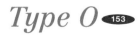

Tomato and Broccoli Ragu NS

2 teaspoons olive oil

1 cup finely diced onions

1 cup finely diced carrots

1 cup finely diced celery

½ cup finely diced parsnips

1 clove garlic, minced

1 cup broccoli florets

3 vine-ripened tomatoes, diced

½ cup Vegetable Stock*

Sea salt, to taste

1 cup Rice Polenta*

¼ cup chopped basil, for garnish

1. Heat olive oil in a large sauté pan over medium heat. Add onion, carrots, celery, and parsnips, and sauté 5 to 6 minutes.

2. Add garlic, broccoli, tomatoes, and stock, and season with sea salt, to taste. Bring to a boil, reduce heat, and simmer for 30 minutes, stirring occasionally.

3. Serve warm on top of Creamy Rice Polenta, and garnish with basil.

*See Vegetable Stock NS recipe (page 223). See Creamy Rice Polenta recipe (page 155).

▶ SERVES 4

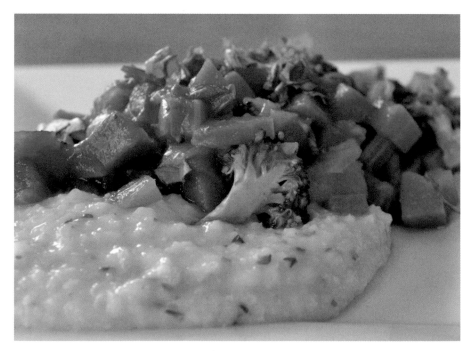

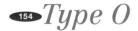

EAT RIGHT FOR YOUR TYPE PERSONALIZED COOKBOOK

½ cup brown rice farina

1 teaspoon dried parsley

¼ cup mozzarella cheese (**NS** substitute manchego cheese or omit cheese)

2 teaspoons olive oil

½ teaspoon onion powder

1. Cook brown rice farina according to package instructions. Two minutes before farina is finished cooking, add remaining ingredients, stirring constantly.

2. Serve immediately.

▶ SERVES 2

tip: If farina is ready before the rest of your meal and becomes too thick, simply add warm water, 1 tablespoon at a time, until desired consistency is achieved.

 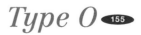

Brown Rice Salad NS

¾ cup brown rice

2 teaspoons olive oil

½ cup diced celery

1 tablespoon sage, chopped

2 cups diced cremini mushrooms

¼ cup finely diced shallots

2 cups arugula

2 tablespoons toasted almonds

1. Cook brown rice according to package instructions. Set aside and let cool slightly.

2. Heat olive oil in a medium skillet over medium heat, and sauté celery, sage, mushrooms, and shallots for 3 to 4 minutes, until vegetables just begin to soften.

3. In a large serving bowl, toss brown rice, mushroom mixture, arugula, and toasted almonds. The warm rice will wilt the arugula slightly.

4. Serve warm or at room temperature.

▶ SERVES 4

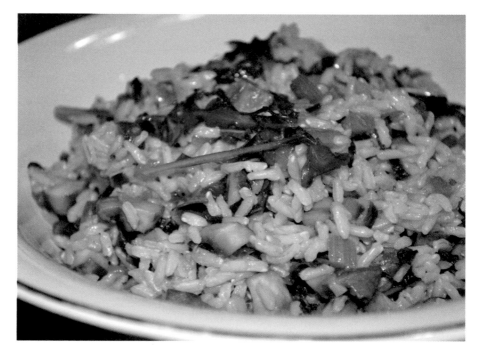

EAT RIGHT FOR YOUR TYPE PERSONALIZED COOKBOOK

Forbidden Black Rice Risotto NS

1. Heat olive oil in a Dutch oven over medium heat. Sauté onion and rice for 3 to 4 minutes, stirring constantly. Season with sea salt.

2. Heat stock and milk in a small saucepan. Add 1 ladle of liquid at a time to the rice and onions, stirring occasionally until liquid is almost absorbed. Repeat until all liquid has been used, 45 minutes.

3. Serve warm.

*See Vegetable Stock NS recipe (page 223).

▶ SERVES 4

2 teaspoons olive oil

½ cup finely diced white onion

1 cup forbidden black rice

½ teaspoon sea salt

2 cups Vegetable Stock*

¾ cup almond milk (NS substitute rice milk)

 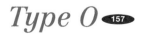

Herbed Quinoa

1 cup quinoa

1 cup Vegetable Stock*

1 cup water

1 tablespoon fresh rosemary

1 tablespoon fresh thyme

1 tablespoon fresh parsley

½ teaspoon lemon zest

2 tablespoons flaxseed

¼ cup crumbled feta cheese (NS omit feta cheese)

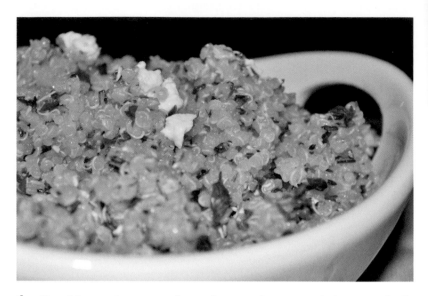

1. Combine quinoa, stock, and water in a pot. Bring to a boil, reduce heat, and simmer for 10 to 12 minutes, until quinoa has absorbed all the water and is soft and tender.

2. Fluff cooked quinoa with a fork, and toss with rosemary, thyme, parsley, lemon zest, flaxseed, and feta cheese.

3. Serve warm.

*See Vegetable Stock NS recipe (page 223).

▶ SERVES 4

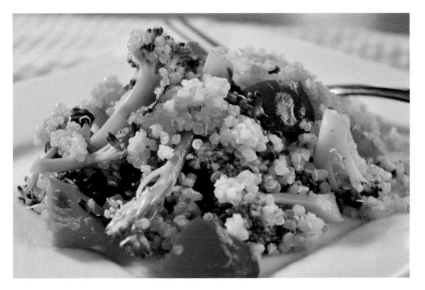

Crisp-Tender Veggie Quinoa NS

1 small head broccoli

1 bunch rappini

1 (4-inch) piece lemongrass

1 cup quinoa

2 cups water

Sea salt, to taste

2 teaspoons olive oil

1 red bell pepper, diced

2 teaspoons lemon zest

1. Chop broccoli and rappini into bite-size pieces. Bring a large pot of water to a boil and cook broccoli and rappini for 3 minutes. Remove with a slotted spoon and place in an ice bath to stop the cooking process. Drain and set aside on a kitchen towel.

2. Bruise lemongrass by hammering with the back of a knife, just until aromatic. Bring quinoa and water to a boil with a pinch of salt, and reduce heat to simmer. Add lemongrass to quinoa and cook 12 minutes.

3. Heat olive oil in a large skillet, and sauté red bell peppers for 3 to 4 minutes. Add broccoli and rappini, and sauté 2 to 3 minutes. Remove lemongrass from cooked quinoa. Add broccoli mixture and lemon zest to quinoa and toss to combine. Season with sea salt, to taste.

4. Serve warm or cold.

▶ SERVES 6

 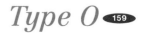

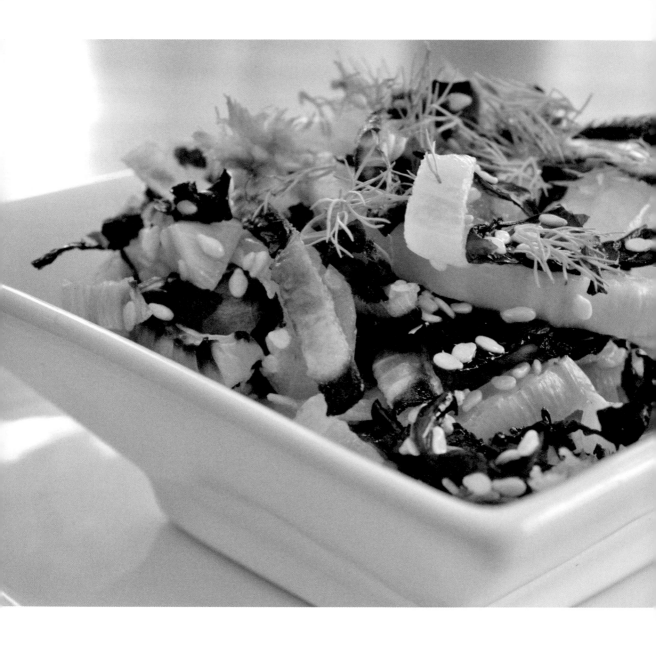

Roasted Wakame and Fennel Salad 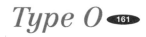NS

1. Preheat oven to 400 degrees.

2. Rinse wakame and place in a bowl of hot water for 5 minutes. Drain and set on paper towels to dry.

3. Trim top and bottom off fennel and discard ends. Cut fennel in half down the center and remove the woody core. Turn fennel cut side down, and slice into thin half-moons. Peel and slice onion into half-moons approximately the same thickness as fennel.

4. Toss fennel, onion, and wakame with olive oil and sprinkle lightly with sea salt. Place in a single layer on a baking sheet, and bake for 15 minutes, until fennel is slightly browned and crispy.

5. Remove baking sheet from the oven, sprinkle with sesame seeds and lemon zest, and bake for an additional 5 minutes.

6. Garnish with dill and serve warm.

▶ **SERVES 4**

2 tablespoons dried wakame

1 bulb fennel

½ yellow onion

1 tablespoon olive oil

Sea salt, to taste

1 tablespoon sesame seeds

2 teaspoons lemon zest

2 tablespoons fresh dill, for garnish

Mint and Cherry Tomato Tabbouleh NS

1 cup quinoa

2 cups water

Sea salt, to taste

3 tablespoons olive oil, divided

4 cups torn kale

1 tablespoon lemon juice

1 tablespoon lemon zest

2 cloves garlic, minced

¾ cup mint

2 cups parsley

1½ cups halved cherry tomatoes

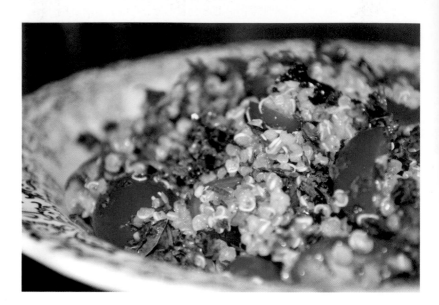

1. Preheat oven to 400 degrees.

2. Combine quinoa, water, and add a dash of sea salt in a saucepan. Bring to a boil, cover, reduce heat, and simmer 10 minutes. Remove from heat, leave covered, and let sit an additional 4 to 5 minutes, until all the water is absorbed and quinoa is tender and fluffy. Fluff with a fork and set aside to cool.

3. Drizzle 2 teaspoons olive oil over kale on a baking sheet and sprinkle with sea salt, to taste. Bake for 10 to 12 minutes until kale pieces are crispy. Remove from oven and set aside.

4. Whisk remaining olive oil, lemon juice, lemon zest, and garlic in a large bowl. Add mint, parsley, tomatoes, quinoa, and kale, and combine until dressing is evenly distributed.

5. Serve at room temperature or chilled.

▶ SERVES 6

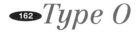
EAT RIGHT FOR YOUR TYPE PERSONALIZED COOKBOOK

Snacks

Toasty Pizza Bites ■ Heirloom Tomato Salsa ■ Crudités and Creamy Goat Cheese Dip S (S Only!) ■ Adzuki Bean Hummus NS ■ Flax Crackers NS ■ Curried Egg Salad NS ■ Farmer Cheese and Beet-Endive Cups ■ Marinated Mozzarella S (S Only!) ■ Spicy Rosemary-Nut Mix ■ Crispy Spring Vegetable Cakes NS ■ Crispy Walnut Bacon–Wrapped Asparagus NS ■ Artichoke Bruschetta ■ Baked Grapefruit ■ Fruit Salad with Mint-Lime Dressing NS ■ Homemade Applesauce ■ Pear and Apple Chips ■ Grilled Pineapple with Cinnamon Syrup ■ Almond Butter Rice Cakes with Mini Chips ■ Carob–Walnut Butter–Stuffed Figs NS

Snacks tend to be the most difficult place for most people to get creative and come up with new ideas that are not overly complicated. Hopefully you'll find in this chapter a few new options to make snacking easier, tastier, and healthier. There are also a few snacks that translate well as appetizers if you like entertaining or have a little extra time to prepare something special.

Toasty Pizza Bites

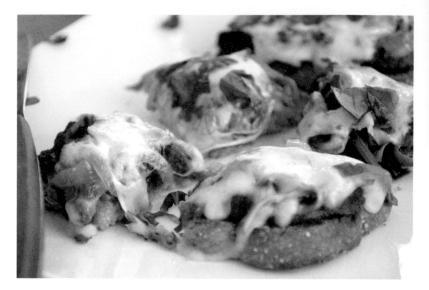

2 teaspoons olive oil

½ cup finely chopped white onion

4 vine-ripened tomatoes, seeded and chopped

1 clove garlic, minced

1 teaspoon agave

Sea salt, to taste

1 tablespoon chopped fresh basil

2 slices gluten-free bread

2 thin slices fresh mozzarella cheese (NS substitute manchego cheese)

½ teaspoon dried oregano

1. Heat olive oil in a large skillet over medium heat, and sauté onion 5 to 6 minutes. Add tomatoes, garlic, and agave, and season with sea salt. Simmer for 8 to 10 minutes, until tomatoes and onion become soft and melt into a slightly thickened sauce. Stir in basil and remove from heat.

2. Lightly toast bread, and top with tomato sauce. Sprinkle with mozzarella cheese and oregano. Place pizza under the broiler for 1 to 2 minutes or until cheese is melted and bubbling, being careful not to let cheese burn.

3. Serve warm.

▶ SERVES 2

1. Bring a large pot of water to a gentle boil. Using a paring knife, make a X on the top of each tomato, place tomatoes into pot, and submerge for up to 1 minute. The skin of the tomato should peel away easily. Dice tomatoes into ½-inch pieces.

2. Heat olive oil in a large skillet over medium heat, and sauté peppers and onion for 6 to 8 minutes. Add garlic and sauté 1 minute. Add tomatoes and cilantro, stir to combine, lower cooking temperature to low and cook for 10 minutes. Season with sea salt. Salsa should be chunky so all vegetables will be tender but retain their shape when done.

3. Remove from heat and let cool completely. Refrigerate and serve chilled.

▶ SERVES 4

4 large heirloom tomatoes

2 teaspoons olive oil

½ cup diced orange bell pepper

½ cup diced red bell pepper

1 large jalapeno, finely diced

1 cup diced white onion

1 garlic clove, minced

¼ cup cilantro (can substitute parsley)

½ teaspoon sea salt

tip: If tomatoes are really ripe, the skin will come off more easily so only keep them in the water for a few seconds. If the tomatoes are not as ripe, it may take 20 seconds, but keep an eye on them so they do not become mushy.

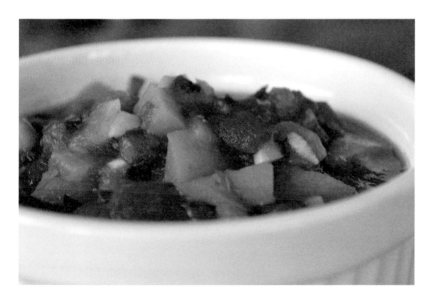

Crudités and Creamy Goat Cheese Dip

dip:

4 ounces soft goat cheese

2 tablespoons chopped dill

2 teaspoons agave

½ teaspoon sea salt

1 tablespoon lemon juice

1 tablespoon almond milk

Baby carrots

Red and orange bell peppers

Kohlrabi sticks

1. Whisk all dip ingredients in a bowl until smooth and seasonings are fully incorporated.

2. Spoon dip into a serving dish, and plate with vegetables.

▶ SERVES 4

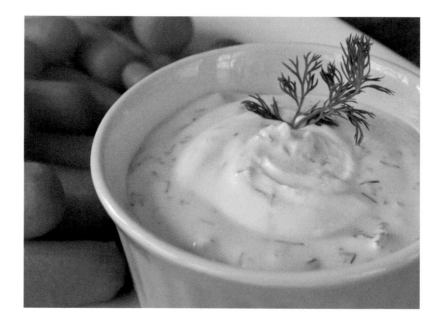

1. Place all ingredients in a food processor or a mini chopper and puree until smooth and creamy.

2. Serve with Flax Crackers NS (page 169) or crudités.

▶ SERVES 4

1½ cups cooked (or canned) adzuki beans, drained and rinsed

½ cup fresh basil, chopped

2 tablespoons fresh parsley, chopped

1 clove garlic, minced

2 teaspoons olive oil

1 tablespoon walnuts

1 teaspoon lemon zest

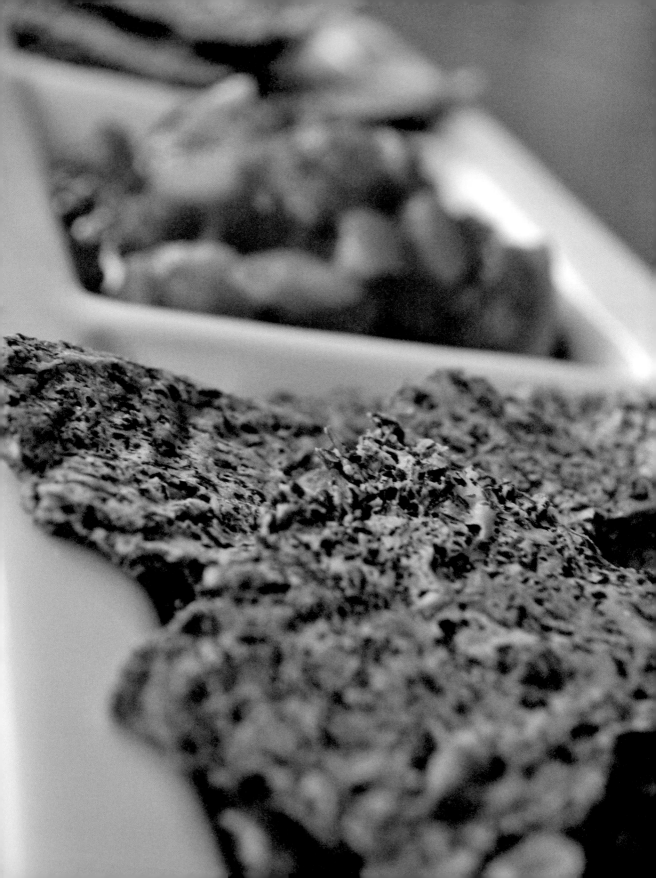

Flax Crackers

1. Combine flaxseed with water, stir, and set aside for 15 minutes, until flax is thick and goopy.

2. Preheat oven to 200 degrees. Line a baking sheet with parchment paper and set aside.

3. Add remaining ingredients to flaxseed, stirring to combine. Mixture will be slightly thicker in consistency than cake batter. Pour flax mixture onto the center of prepared baking sheet. Spray an offset spatula with cooking spray or coat with olive oil to help you spread the flax mixture without sticking. Spread the mixture in an even layer, as thin as possible, across the whole baking sheet.

4. Bake for 2 hours, until crackers solidify and are slightly rubbery in texture.

5. Increase oven temperature to 400 degrees, and bake 10 minutes. Carefully flip the crackers, and bake an additional 5 to 6 minutes. When done, crackers will be hardened and crispy on both sides. Let cool, and break apart into pieces the size of tortilla chips. Serve room temperature, and store in a cool, dry place or in the freezer.

▶ **SERVES 4**

1 cup coarsely ground flaxseed

⅔ cup hot water

¼ teaspoon sea salt

¼ cup pepitas (pumpkin seeds)

3 tablespoons almond flour

tip: Whole flax seeds will last longer than ground, so buy whole, and grind in a coffee grinder or food processor when needed to maximize shelf life.

 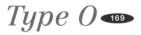

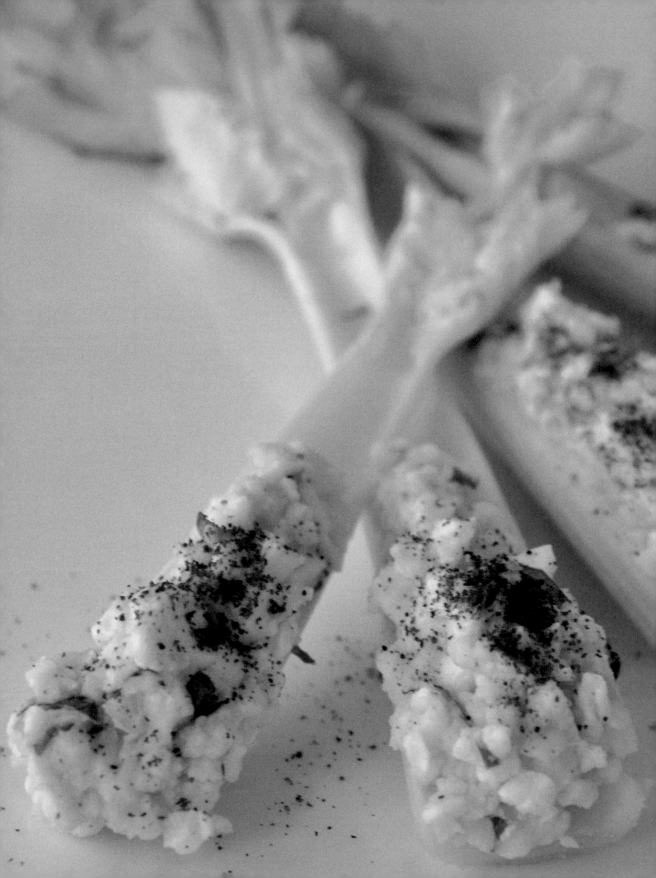

Curried Egg Salad NS

1. Place eggs in a saucepan, and cover with cold water. Bring to a boil, and turn off the heat. Set a timer for 14 minutes, and when done, rinse eggs under cold water. Peel eggs, chop, and place them in a large bowl.

2. Add remaining ingredients to the bowl, and toss to combine.

3. Serve on celery sticks or between two pieces of brown rice toast.

▶ SERVES 4

4 large eggs

½ teaspoon dried mustard

1 tablespoon chopped parsley

¼ teaspoon sea salt

½ teaspoon curry powder

⅛ teaspoon turmeric

2 teaspoons olive oil

2 teaspoons lemon juice

 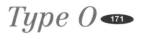

Farmer Cheese and Beet-Endive Cups

2 medium orange beets

2 medium red beets

2 teaspoons olive oil

¼ cup farmer cheese (NS omit farmer cheese)

¼ cup chopped walnuts

1 teaspoon lemon juice

Sea salt, to taste

2 heads endive

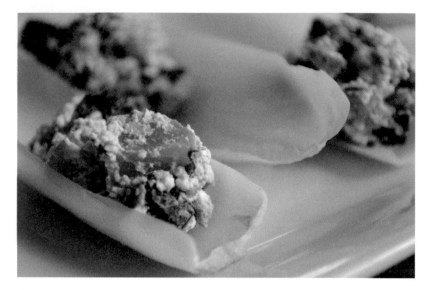

1. Preheat oven to 400 degrees. Line a baking sheet with tinfoil and set aside.

2. Trim tops and bottoms off beets and scrub clean. Place on prepared baking sheet, drizzle with olive oil, and bake for 60 to 65 minutes or until easily pierced with a knife.

3. Let beets cool for 10 minutes. Carefully remove skin with a paring knife, and dice into ½-inch cubes. Place in a bowl with cheese, walnuts, and lemon juice. (NS, toss beets with walnuts, lemon juice, 1 tablespoon olive oil, and 1 teaspoon fresh sage, and continue with recipe.) Season with sea salt, to taste, and toss to combine.

4. Spoon 2 teaspoons filling onto each endive leaf. Serve immediately or chill, covered, in the refrigerator until ready to serve.

► SERVES 4

tip: Store-bought, precooked beets, either canned or in vacuum-sealed packages in the produce department can be substituted in this recipe, but beets from a can tend to lose a great deal of flavor and sweetness.

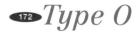

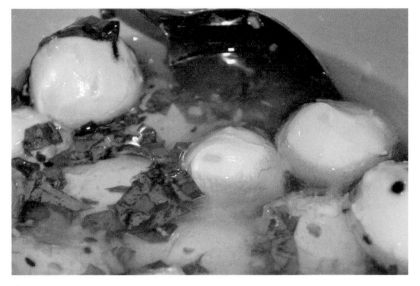

½ cup extra virgin olive oil

1 teaspoon large-grain sea salt

1 teaspoon crushed red pepper

2 cloves garlic, minced

2 tablespoons chopped basil

2 finely diced green olives

1 pound fresh mozzarella balls

1. Place olive oil, sea salt, crushed red pepper, garlic, basil, and olives in a medium-size bowl, stirring to incorporate. Add mozzarella balls, toss to coat, and refrigerate for at least 2 hours.

2. Remove from refrigerator 15 minutes before serving to allow oil to come to room temperature.

3. Marinated mozzarella will keep in refrigerator for up to 1 week.

▶ **SERVES 4**

tip: If you cannot find individually portioned miniature mozzarella balls, buy 1 large ball of fresh cheese and cut into 1–2-inch pieces.

Spicy Rosemary-Nut Mix

2 tablespoons fresh chopped rosemary

1 teaspoon red chili powder

½ teaspoon salt

1 tablespoon maple syrup (NS substitute agave)

2 teaspoons ghee

1 cup quartered black or English walnuts

½ cup roughly chopped pecans

½ cup crushed almonds

1. Preheat oven to 325 degrees.

2. Toss all ingredients in a bowl and spread on a baking sheet. Bake 25 minutes, tossing halfway through. Nuts will be aromatic and lightly browned when done. Let cool and spoon into a bowl to serve.

3. Store in a cool, dry place for up to 1 week.

▶ SERVES 6

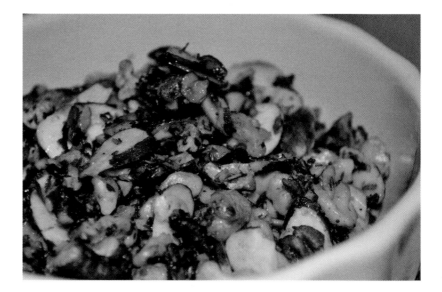

EAT RIGHT FOR YOUR TYPE PERSONALIZED COOKBOOK

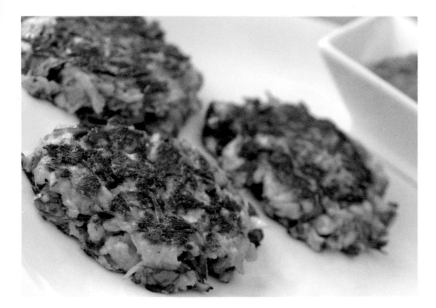

Crispy Spring Vegetable Cakes NS

1 small celeriac (celery root), peeled

1 small bulb fennel

2 tablespoons grated onion

2 cups spinach

½ teaspoon lemon zest

1 tablespoon chopped sage

1 large egg

2 tablespoons brown rice flour

⅓ cup bread crumbs*

2 teaspoons olive oil

1. Use a food processor or a hand grater to shred celeriac and fennel. Place vegetables and onion in a bowl. Finely chop spinach and add to vegetables with lemon zest, sage, egg, flour, and bread crumbs. Toss to combine.

2. Heat olive oil in a large skillet over medium heat. Using an ice cream scoop, spoon vegetable mixture into a large frying pan, leaving 1 inch between each cake. Cook 2 to 3 minutes, turn, and cook an additional 2 to 3 minutes, until cakes are brown and crispy on each side and warm and tender in the center.

3. Serve warm.

*See Basic Gluten-Free Bread Crumbs NS recipe (page 224).

▶ SERVES 4

tip: Cool and refrigerate vegetable cakes to eat for a snack, or for breakfast topped with a poached or fried egg.

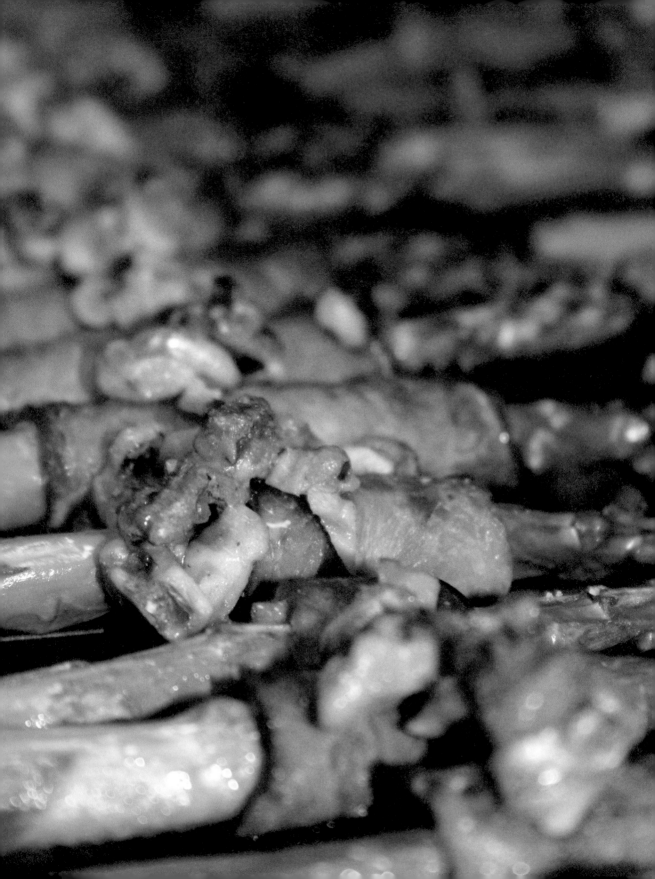

Crispy Walnut Bacon–Wrapped Asparagus NS

1. Preheat oven to 375 degrees. Grease a wire baking rack with nonstick cooking spray and set aside.

2. Combine maple syrup, ginger, and walnuts in a small bowl, and set aside.

3. Cut off and discard woody bottoms of asparagus. Toss spears with olive oil. Slice bacon lengthwise and then into thirds. Wrap bacon around each spear of asparagus, and place on prepared rack. Repeat with remaining asparagus and bacon.

4. Place wire rack on a baking sheet. Spoon the maple-walnut mixture over asparagus.

5. Bake 10 to 12 minutes on center oven rack, until walnuts begin to smell nutty and edges of bacon are crispy.

6. Serve warm.

▶ SERVES 6

2 tablespoons maple syrup

1 teaspoon ground ginger

½ cup chopped walnuts

1 bunch asparagus spears

5 slices turkey bacon

2 teaspoons olive oil

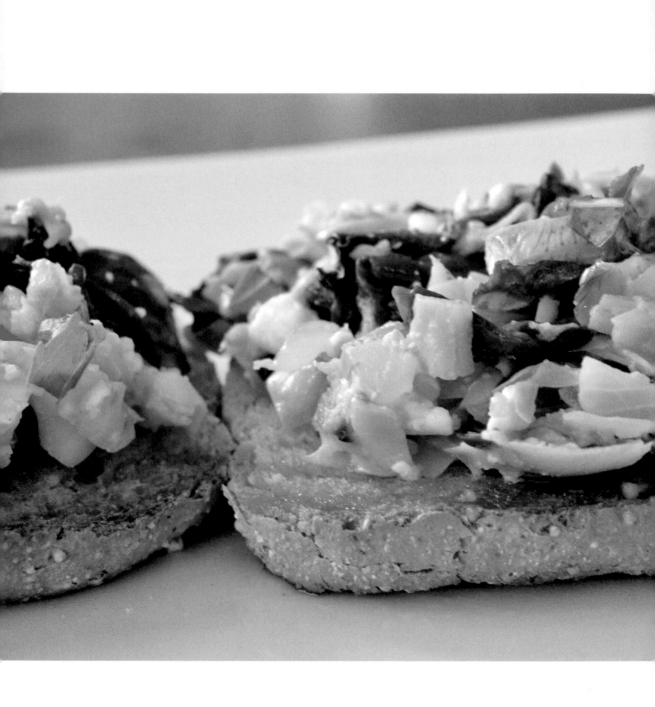

Artichoke Bruschetta

1. Heat 2 teaspoons olive oil in medium skillet over medium heat, and sauté artichokes and onion, 4 to 5 minutes. Season with sea salt and add spinach; sauté an additional 2 to 3 minutes, until spinach is wilted and artichokes are tender and hot.

2. While the vegetables cook, lightly toast the bread and rub toast with halved garlic. Drizzle toast evenly with remaining 1 teaspoon olive oil.

3. Remove vegetables from heat, and mix in feta cheese. Spoon mixture evenly over toast, and serve warm or at room temperature.

▶ SERVES 2

1 tablespoon olive oil, divided

1 cup frozen artichoke hearts, thawed and chopped

¼ cup finely diced onions

¼ teaspoon sea salt

2 cups chopped spinach

3 slices brown rice/millet bread

1 clove garlic, halved

¼ cup feta cheese, crumbled (NS omit feta cheese)

 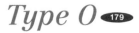

Baked Grapefruit

2 whole ruby red
grapefruits, halved

2 teaspoons honey

½ teaspoon cinnamon (NS
omit cinnamon)

1. Preheat oven to 400 degrees.

2. Trim the rounded bottom of each grapefruit half to create a stable base. Place on a baking sheet, cut flesh side up.

3. Drizzle each half evenly with honey and cinnamon.

4. Bake for 5 to 6 minutes, then broil for 1 to 2 additional minutes until the edges of the grapefruit are browned and the fruit is hot and the top is bubbling.

▶ **SERVES 4**

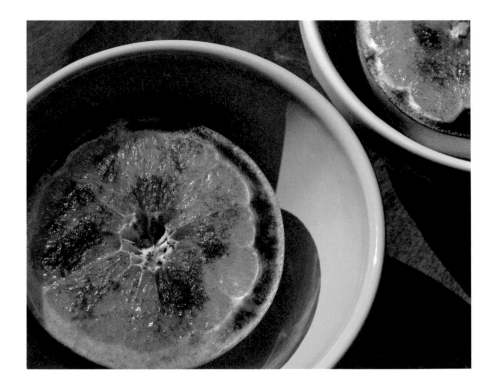

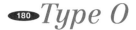

1. Place dried cranberries in a small bowl. Cover with hot water and steep for 10 minutes, to rehydrate.

2. Dice peaches, pineapple, and mango into ½-inch pieces, and toss in a large serving bowl with cherries.

3. Drain cranberries, and gently pat dry on a kitchen towel.

4. Whisk lime zest, juice, agave, and mint leaves in a small bowl, and pour over fruit salad. Top with cranberries, toss, and serve chilled.

▶ SERVES 6

½ cup dried cranberries
2 organic peaches
1 pineapple
2 organic mangoes
2 cups fresh cherries, pitted and quartered
Zest and juice of 2 limes
1 teaspoon agave
½ cup finely chopped mint leaves

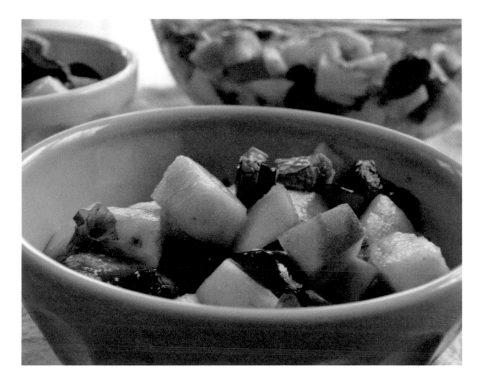

Homemade Applesauce

2 Red Delicious organic apples (about 2 cups diced) (NS substitute Bosc pears)

2 Granny Smith organic apples (about 2 cups diced) (NS substitute Bosc pears)

1 cinnamon stick (NS omit cinnamon)

½ cup apple juice (NS substitute pear juice)

½ cup frozen or fresh organic cranberries

1–2 tablespoons agave

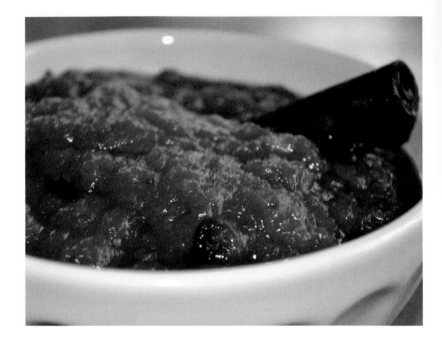

1. Combine apples, cinnamon stick, apple juice, and cranberries in a saucepan set over medium heat. Add 1 tablespoon agave to start; add up to 1 additional tablespoon depending on tartness of apples and cranberries. Cook 30 minutes, or until apples no longer hold their shape.

2. Stir occasionally, remove from heat, and serve warm or chilled.

▶ **SERVES 6**

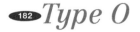

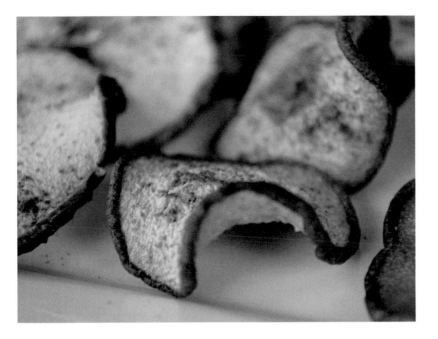

Pear and Apple Chips

2 Bosc pears

2 Bartlett pears

2 Braeburn apples (NS substitute pears)

¼ teaspoon cinnamon (NS omit cinnamon)

1. Preheat oven to 225 degrees. Line two baking sheets with parchment paper and set aside.

2. Slice pears and apples in rounds as thinly as you can, or use a mandolin to help you. Place fruit in a single layer on prepared baking sheets and sprinkle evenly with cinnamon.

3. Bake for 2 hours, flipping fruit halfway through cooking.

4. Cool completely, and serve.

▶ SERVES 4

Grilled Pineapple with Cinnamon Syrup

2 teaspoons light olive oil

1 fresh pineapple

¼ cup Cinnamon Syrup* (NS substitute agave or Chocolate Syrup*)

1. Preheat grill pan over medium heat and brush with oil to create a nonstick surface. Remove outer layer of pineapple, core, and slice into rounds.

2. Brush 1 side of pineapple rounds with Cinnamon Syrup and place sauce side down on the grill pan. Cook 2 to 3 minutes, and brush the opposite side with Cinnamon Syrup.

3. Flip, and grill an additional 2 to 3 minutes.

4. Serve warm.

*See Cinnamon Syrup recipe (page 220). **NS**, see Chocolate Syrup **NS** recipe (page 219).

▶ **SERVES 4**

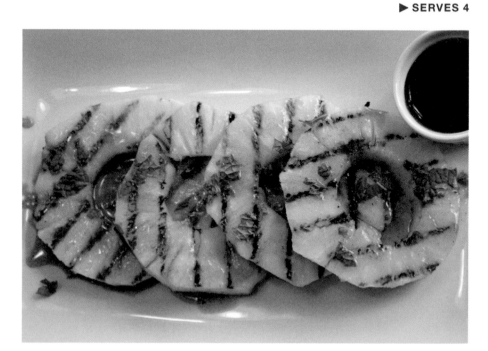

EAT RIGHT FOR YOUR TYPE PERSONALIZED COOKBOOK

Almond Butter Rice Cakes with Mini Chips

1. Spread 2 tablespoons almond butter on each rice cake, and top each with slices from ½ banana, 1 tablespoon chocolate chips, and ½ teaspoon honey.

▶ SERVES 2

4 tablespoons almond butter

2 rice cakes

1 banana

2 tablespoons mini dark chocolate chips

1 teaspoon honey (NS substitute agave)

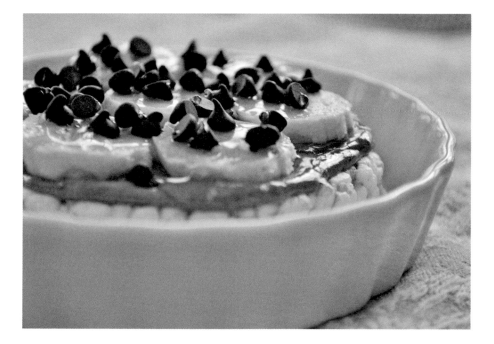

Carob–Walnut Butter–Stuffed Figs 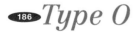 NS

5 fresh or dried figs

¼ cup walnut halves

2 tablespoons pecans

1 tablespoon Carob Extract™ plus more for garnish*

1 teaspoon olive oil

3 tablespoons hot water

Sea salt, to taste

1. Slice figs in half from stem to base, and set aside.

2. In a food processor, combine walnuts, pecans, Carob Extract™, and olive oil and pulse to combine. With the processor running, drizzle in hot water so that the mixture forms a thick paste similar in consistency to natural peanut butter. Season with salt, to taste.

3. Spoon about 1 teaspoon nut butter mixture over each fig half, and drizzle with additional Carob Extract™, if desired.

▶ SERVES 2

*Information about purchasing Carob Extract™ can be found in Appendix II: Products (page 249).

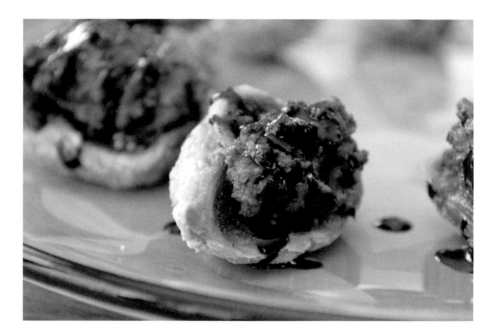

EAT RIGHT FOR YOUR TYPE PERSONALIZED COOKBOOK

Drinks and Beverages

Cooling Chamomile Spritzer NS ■ *Cherry Spritzer* NS ■ *Carrot, Kale, and Ginger Juice* ■ *Sweet Basil and Ginger Tea* NS ■ *Mango-Kale Smoothie* ■ *Matcha-Mojito Tea* ■ *Creamy Banana–Nut Butter Smoothie* ■ *Pineapple Spa Water* NS ■ *Berry Bonanza Smoothie*

Any time you start a new diet plan, it is nice to have as many taste and flavor options available to you, especially when you are just getting started. These will help to add diversity to your day in simple and tasty ways. There are plenty of us who have a routine of drinking coffee, black tea, or soda, and the following beverage suggestions can help to substitute for the old habits you are trying to kick. Also included in this chapter are recipes for smoothies, which can spice up your snack or breakfast routine or maybe even replace that milk shake that becomes tempting in the hot, summer months.

Cooling Chamomile Spritzer NS

4 cups water
½ cup sliced peaches
1 cup mint leaves
4 chamomile tea bags
2 cups sparkling water
¼ cup peach nectar

1. Bring water to a gentle boil, and remove from heat. Add peaches, mint leaves, and tea bags, and steep for 4 to 5 minutes. Remove tea bags, and cool in refrigerator until chilled, about 1 hour. Add sparkling water and peach nectar, and stir.

2. Serve over ice.

▶ SERVES 4

Cherry Spritzer NS

6 pitted cherries
½ cup mint leaves
½ cup black cherry juice
1 pint seltzer water

1. In the bottom of a large pitcher, crush cherries and mint leaves. Add cherry juice and seltzer, and stir to combine.

2. Serve over ice.

▶ SERVES 4

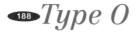

1 bunch kale

½ lemon

4 large carrots

4 apples (NS substitute pears)

1 (3-inch) piece fresh ginger, peeled

1. Wash and dry vegetables. Cut off tough ends of the kale and carrots, and push kale, lemon, carrots, apples, and ginger through juicer one at a time. Stir together and enjoy.

▶ SERVES 4

tip: Vegetable juices will keep in the refrigerator for up to 3 days, but provide the best nutritional value when consumed immediately after juicing.

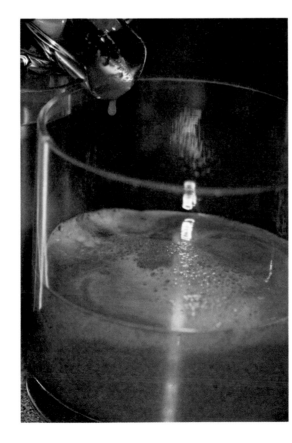

 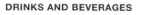

Sweet Basil and Ginger Tea (NS)

4 cups water

1 (2-inch) piece ginger, peeled and roughly chopped

¼ cup torn basil leaves

1 teaspoon agave nectar

1. Bring water to a boil with ginger, remove from heat, and add basil leaves. Let steep at least 3 minutes. Stir in agave.

2. Serve warm.

▶ SERVES 2

Mango-Kale Smoothie

1 cup diced, frozen mango

¼ cup frozen pineapple

½ frozen banana

¼ cup frozen kale

¾ cup almond milk (NS substitute rice milk)

2 teaspoons agave

2 tablespoons Protein Blend Powder™—Type O*

½ teaspoon ground cinnamon

1. Place all ingredients in a blender and blend until smooth. Or, place all ingredients in a large cup and blend with an immersion blender.

▶ SERVES 4

*Information about purchasing Protein Blend™ Powder—Type O can be found in Appendix II: Products (page 249).

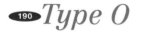

Matcha-Mojito Tea

1. Heat water until almost at a boil. Add mint and lime zest and juice, and let steep, covered, for 5 minutes.

2. Spoon matcha powder into a heat-safe glass pitcher and gradually pour minty water over the matcha, whisking continuously. Strain the mint and zest out of the tea. Add honey and serve.

▶ **SERVES 4**

6 cups water

1 cup fresh mint

Zest and juice of 1 lime

2 teaspoons matcha powder

1 tablespoon honey (NS substitute agave)

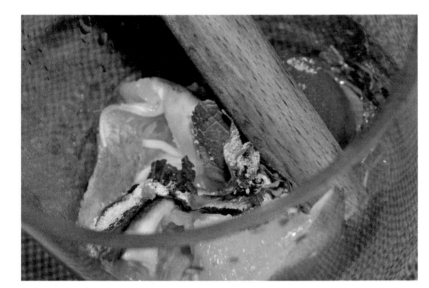

 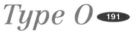

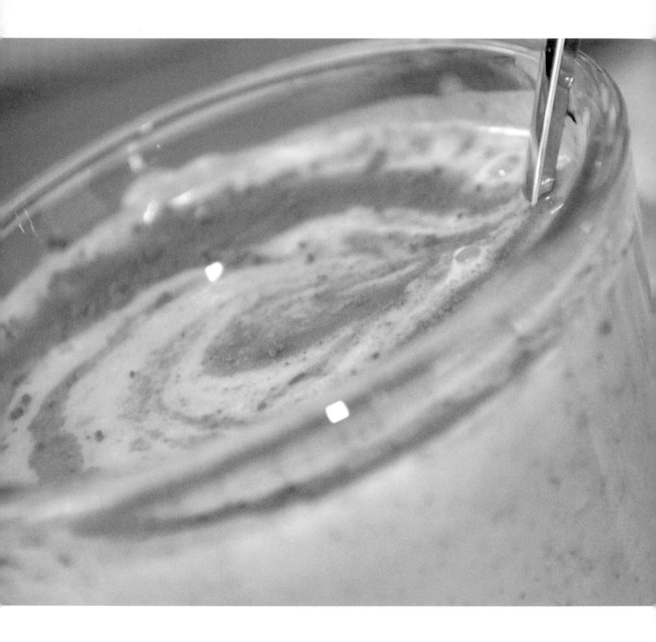

1. Combine all ingredients in a food processor and puree, or use an immersion blender. For easier blending, add liquid to the food processor first.

▶ SERVES 2

*Information about purchasing Protein Blend™ Powder—Type O can be found in Appendix II: Products (page 249).

1 frozen banana

1 teaspoon agave

2 tablespoons Protein Blend Powder™— Type O*

1 cup almond milk (NS substitute rice milk)

¼ cup frozen mango

1 tablespoon flaxseed

1½ tablespoons almond butter

 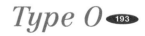

Pineapple Spa Water (NS)

2 sprigs mint

6 cup water

4 (¼-inch-thick) pineapple slices

1. Wash mint and place in a large pitcher with water and pineapple slices. Let chill in refrigerator for 2 to 3 hours.

2. Serve chilled.

▶ SERVES 4

Berry Bonanza Smoothie

½ cup raspberries

½ cup pineapple

¾ cup blueberries

1 cup torn kale

1 cup almond milk (NS substitute rice milk)

2 tablespoons almond butter

2 teaspoons agave

1 tablespoon flaxseed

2 scoops Protein Blend Powder™—Type O*

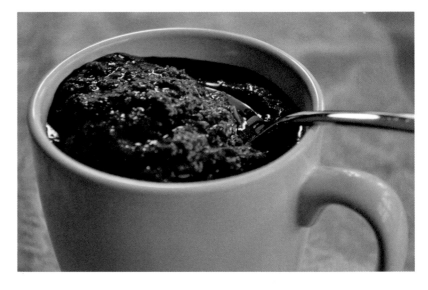

1. Combine all ingredients in a blender and blend until smooth. Pour into two glasses and serve cold.

▶ SERVES 2

*Information about purchasing Protein Blend™ Powder—Type O can be found in Appendix II: Products (page 249).

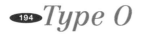

Desserts

Deep-Chocolate Brownies ■ *Chocolate Salted-Nut Clusters* NS ■ *Chocolate Chip Cookies* ■ *Cocoa-Dusted Chocolate Truffles* ■ *Almond-Cranberry Biscotti* ■ *Fig Bars* ■ *Blueberry Crumble* ■ *Peach-Cinnamon Charlotte* ■ *Carrot-Pineapple Cake with Chocolate-Chai Frosting* ■ *Upside-Down Almond Cake with Apricot Glaze* ■ *Matcha Cake with Chocolate Frosting* ■ *Crêpes with Raspberry Chutney (S)* NS ■ *Banana-Based Ice Cream: 4 Ways* ■ *Ginger Rice Pudding*

What is a cookbook without desserts? The best way to stick to any kind of diet is to have realistic options for indulging your sweet tooth once in a while. Although these recipes sound indulgent, they are written to be as healthful as possible while still feeling like satisfying desserts. Whenever possible, use agave or molasses as sweeteners, include allowable grains, limit fats, and feel free to use chocolate.

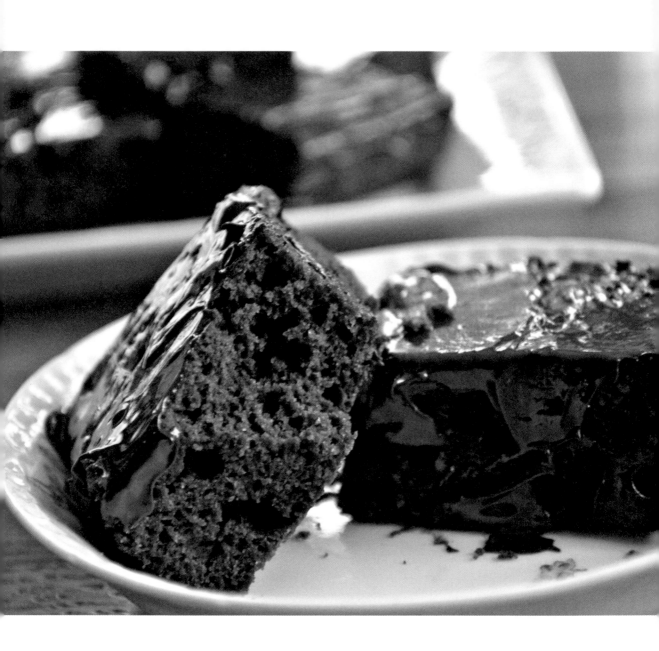

Deep-Chocolate Brownies

1. Preheat oven to 350 degrees. Grease an 8" x 8" baking dish with nonstick cooking spray and set aside.

2. In a large bowl, combine flours, arrowroot starch, cocoa powder, and sea salt. Set aside.

3. Place shaved chocolate in a small bowl, and whisk in warm water until chocolate fully melts, adding 1 more tablespoon water if necessary, and set aside.

4. Whisk eggs, applesauce, butter, and agave in a medium bowl. Add to dry ingredients, and stir to combine. Once combined, add melted chocolate and stir to incorporate.

5. Pour into prepared baking dish, and bake for 30 minutes or until a cake tester or toothpick inserted in brownies comes out clean.

6. Remove brownies from the oven, and turn off heat. Pour chocolate chips over the top of the brownies, and place back into the oven for 2 to 3 minutes. Use an offset spatula to spread melted chips evenly across the top of the brownies. Let cool 10 minutes.

7. Slice and serve. Brownies will stay in a cool, dry place overnight or in the freezer for up to 1 month.

▶ SERVES 8

*Ghee or light olive oil can be substituted here.

⅔ cup brown rice flour

⅓ cup millet flour

⅓ cup arrowroot starch

3 tablespoons cocoa powder

½ teaspoon sea salt

2 ounces 100 percent dark chocolate, shaved

3 tablespoons warm water

3 large eggs

¼ cup applesauce (NS substitute ½ smashed banana)

4 tablespoons butter, softened*

½ cup agave

½ cup chocolate chips

Chocolate Salted-Nut Clusters (NS)

1 cup whole almonds

½ cup quartered walnuts

½ cup halved macadamia nuts

2 teaspoons blackstrap molasses

1 teaspoon agave

½ cup chocolate chips

1 teaspoon large-grain sea salt

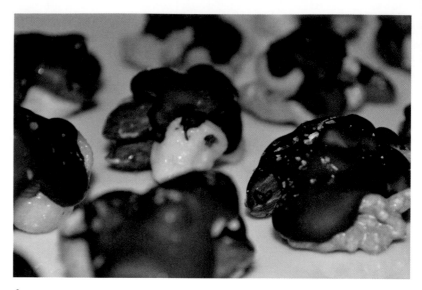

1. Preheat oven to 350 degrees.

2. Place almonds, walnuts, and macadamia nuts in a medium bowl, and toss to combine.

3. In a small saucepan, heat molasses and agave for 30 seconds over medium-low heat, just until melted. Drizzle over nuts and toss. Very gently, spoon about 1 tablespoon of the nut clusters onto a wire cooling rack (if you do not have one, you can spoon the same amount into mini cupcake pans coated with nonstick spray). Place wire rack in the oven and bake for 8 to 10 minutes.

4. Remove and let cool. Once cool, place in freezer for at least 10 minutes.

5. Melt chocolate chips over a double boiler, being careful not to let water in double boiler touch base of the top pan.

6. Remove nut clusters from the freezer, spoon melted chocolate over the top, sprinkle evenly with sea salt, and freeze for 10 minutes.

7. Serve cold or room temperature. Keep in an airtight glass container for up to 1 week, or freeze for 1 month.

▶ SERVES 6

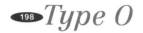

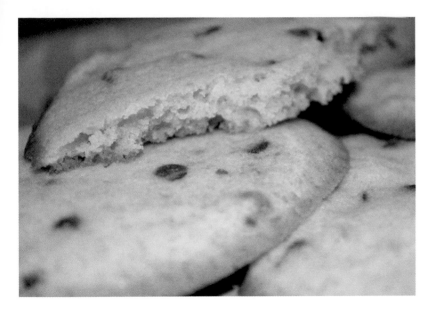

Chocolate Chip Cookies

¾ cup brown rice flour

½ cup millet flour

¼ cup arrowroot starch

2 teaspoons baking powder

1 teaspoon sea salt

½ cup (1 stick) butter, softened (NS substitute ½ cup ghee)

½ cup agave

2 tablespoons blackstrap molasses

1 large egg

1 large egg white

½ cup allergy-free chocolate chips

1. Preheat oven to 350 degrees. Line an 18-inch baking sheet with parchment paper and set aside.

2. In a large bowl, mix flours with arrowroot starch, baking powder, and salt, and set aside.

3. In a separate bowl, beat softened butter with agave and molasses until smooth and creamy. Add egg and egg white, beating slightly.

4. Add egg mixture to flour mixture and stir just until combined and free of lumps. Stir in chocolate chips.

5. Spoon dough by the tablespoonful, 2 inches apart on prepared baking sheet.

6. Bake 12 minutes in the center rack of the oven, until cookies are golden brown around the edges and soft in the center. Let cool on a wire rack or eat warm.

7. Store in an airtight container in a cool, dry place for 1 to 2 days, or in the freezer for up to 1 month.

▶ SERVES 12

 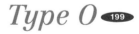

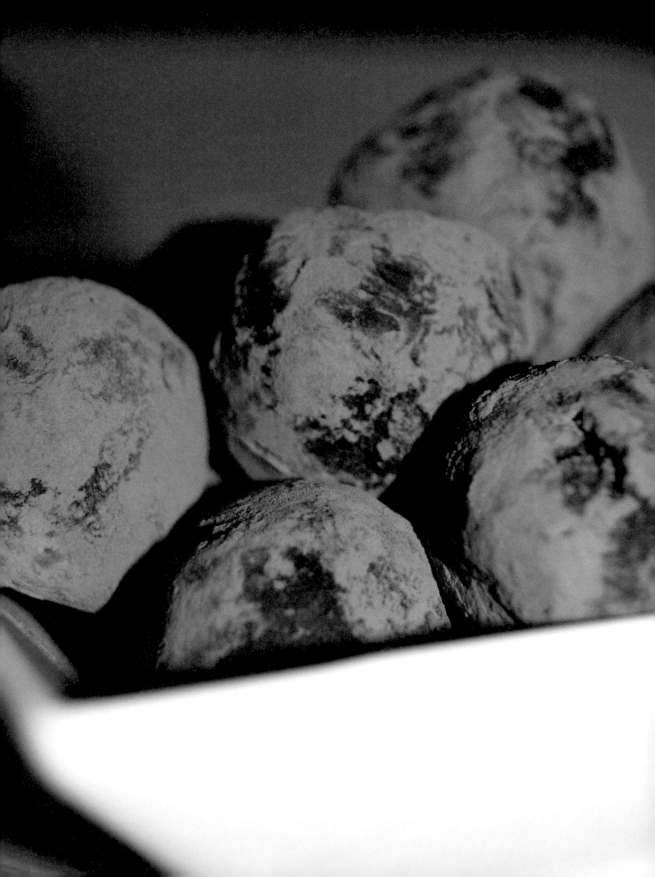

Cocoa-Dusted Chocolate Truffles

1. Shave chocolate and place in a medium bowl. Warm butter, agave nectar, milk, and salt in a saucepan set over medium heat. Pour mixture over chocolate, whisking continuously until smooth.

2. Cool mixture to room temperature, then cover tightly and refrigerate until chocolate is firm, about 2 to 3 hours.

3. Using a tablespoon or melon baller, scoop out truffles and roll into balls slightly smaller than a golf ball, then gently roll around in cocoa powder. Refrigerate until serving.

4. Store in an airtight container in the refrigerator for up to 1 week.

▶ SERVES 6

8 ounces 100 percent dark chocolate

¼ cup butter

⅔ cup agave nectar

½ cup almond milk (NS substitute rice milk)

⅛ teaspoon large-grain sea salt

3 tablespoons cocoa powder

featured ingredient

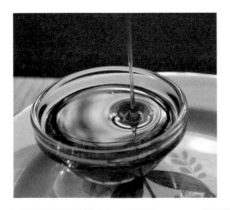

agave nectar

Agave is a natural sweetener derived from the agave plant, commonly found in the southwestern United States and in Mexico. Agave is most well-known for its role as the base ingredient of tequila. It can be used in baking and cooking in place of sugar; however, because it is a liquid, the agave-to-sugar ratio is not 1:1. Agave has a mild taste akin to that of honey, but its flavor is much less noticeable.

 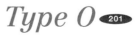

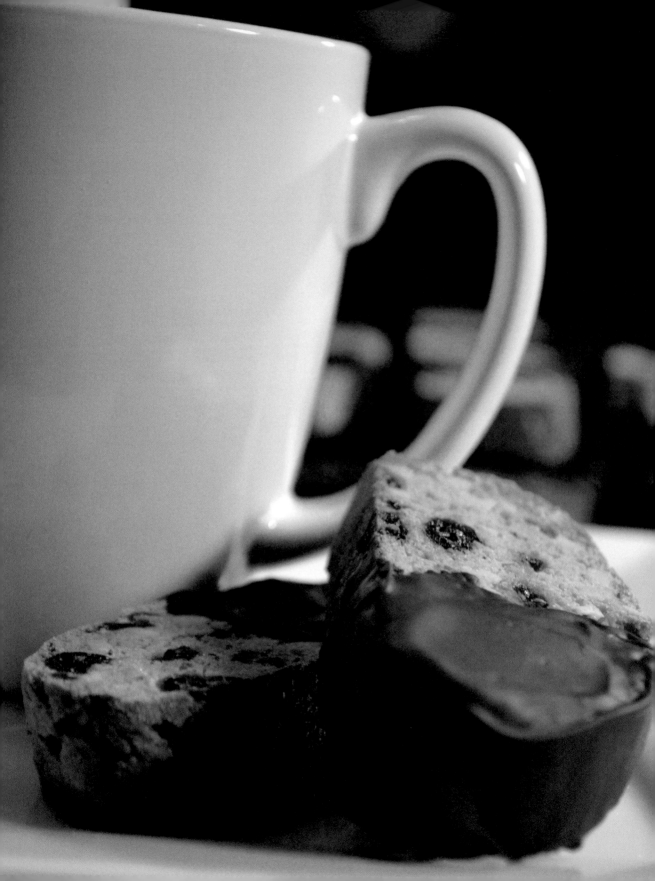

Almond-Cranberry Biscotti

1. Preheat oven to 350 degrees. Line an 11" x 17" baking sheet with parchment paper and set aside.

2. Place cranberries in a small bowl and cover with hot water to rehydrate; let steep for 10 minutes.

3. In a large bowl, mix together flours, baking powder, salt, and almonds.

4. In a separate bowl, whisk eggs, lemon zest, agave, and apricot jam. Add egg mixture to dry ingredients, stirring just until combined. Drain cranberries, pat dry, and add to dough.

5. Gather dough into a ball, and place on floured work surface. Using your hands, gently roll into a long, flat log the length of your baking sheet. Place on prepared baking sheet and bake for 30 minutes. Remove from oven and let cool 5 minutes. At this point, the cookie will have the texture of soft bread. Cut biscotti on the bias into ¾-inch slices, using a serrated knife. Place each section flat on the baking sheet, and bake for an additional 25 minutes, flipping once halfway through baking to ensure cookies are dry and crunchy all the way through.

6. Remove from oven, and let cool on a drying rack. If using chocolate, heat chocolate morsels over a double boiler until melted and silky. Spoon chocolate over half of each cooled biscotti, and let the chocolate cool again.

7. Serve at room temperature. Store in a cool, dry place overnight or in the freezer for up to 1 month.

▶ SERVES 12

¾ cup dried cranberries

1 cup amaranth flour

1½ cups brown rice flour plus more for rolling

3 teaspoons baking powder

½ teaspoon fine-grain sea salt

1 cup slivered almonds

3 large eggs

1 teaspoon lemon zest

⅓ cup agave

⅓ cup apricot jam (NS substitute cherry jam)

½ cup allergy-free chocolate morsels (optional)

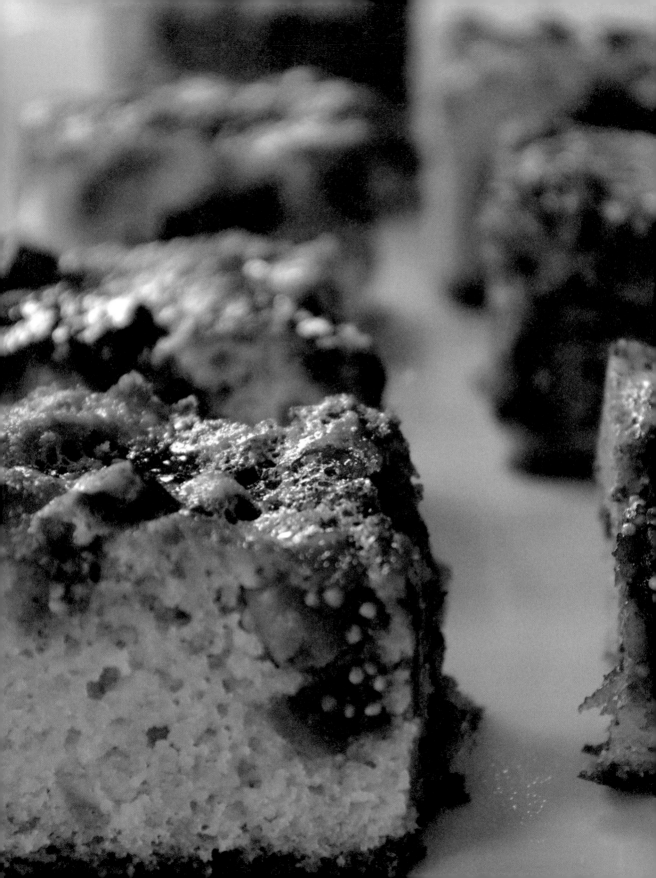

Fig Bars

1. Preheat oven to 350 degrees. Grease an 9" x 11" baking dish with ghee and set aside.

2. Combine flours with baking powder and sea salt in a large bowl. Mix just until combined.

3. Whisk eggs with cooled ghee, and add to flour mixture, mixing until smooth and free of lumps.

4. In a clean, dry, glass bowl, beat egg whites until they form stiff peaks. Fold egg whites into batter, one-third at a time.

5. Pour batter into prepared baking dish, and bake for about 15 minutes, until crust begins to firm.

6. While crust cooks, combine all topping ingredients in a medium bowl, mixing until well combined.

7. Remove crust from oven and spoon topping mixture evenly over top. Return to the oven and bake an additional 35 to 40 minutes or until a cake tester comes out clean.

8. Serve warm or room temperature. Bars will stay in a cool, dry place for 1 to 2 days or freeze for up to 1 month.

▶ SERVES 12

⅔ cup brown rice flour

¼ cup millet flour

¼ cup arrowroot flour

1 teaspoon baking powder

½ teaspoon sea salt

2 large eggs

4 tablespoons ghee, melted and cooled, plus more for greasing

2 large egg whites

topping:

½ cup fig jam

½ cup dried figs, cut into ½-inch dice

¼ cup agave

2 eggs, slightly beaten

1 egg white

2 teaspoons lemon zest

½ teaspoon ground cinnamon (NS substitute ¼ teaspoon ginger and ⅛ teaspoon nutmeg)

⅛ teaspoon ground cloves

2 tablespoons brown rice flour

Blueberry Crumble

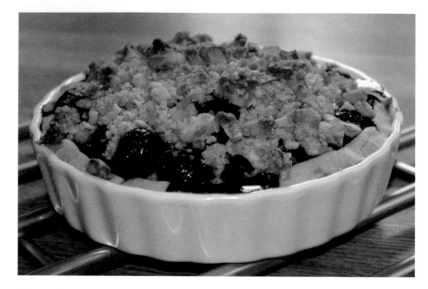

crust:

⅓ cup tapioca flour (NS substitute arrowroot starch)

⅔ cup brown rice flour plus extra for rolling

½ teaspoon sea salt

3 tablespoons cold butter

4–5 tablespoons ice water

filling:

1 teaspoon lemon zest

¼ teaspoon sea salt

¼ teaspoon ground cinnamon (NS substitute ⅛ teaspoon nutmeg)

⅓ cup agave

¼ teaspoon ground ginger

2 cups (fresh or frozen) blueberries

topping:

¼ cup finely chopped walnuts

¼ cup brown rice flour

2 tablespoons cold butter or ghee

1 tablespoon agave

1. Preheat oven to 350 degrees.

2. Combine flours and sea salt in a large bowl. Cut cold butter into small pieces and add to flour mixture. Using a crossing motion with two butter knives or a pastry cutter, incorporate butter into the flour until the mixture resembles coarse cornmeal. Add water, 1 tablespoon at a time, until the dough comes together but is not sticky. Gather dough in a ball and knead until it becomes smooth and pliable, using more flour if needed. Small pieces of butter should still be visible. Cover dough and refrigerate 1 hour.

3. On a floured surface, roll dough into a 12-inch circle. Carefully lift into an 8-inch pie dish, using a spatula to help you. (If dough rips, simply press back together.)

4. Stir together filling ingredients in a large bowl, just until combined, and spoon into pie crust.

5. Combine walnuts and brown rice flour in a large bowl. Incorporate butter into mixture using your fingers. Stir in agave, and sprinkle on top of blueberry filling.

6. Bake for 25 to 30 minutes.

▶ SERVES 4

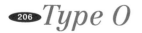

EAT RIGHT FOR YOUR TYPE PERSONALIZED COOKBOOK

1. Preheat oven to 350 degrees. Grease 2 (12-oz.) ramekins with ghee, and set aside.

2. Heat ghee and olive oil in a large skillet over medium heat. Add peaches, cranberries, and walnuts, and cook 5 minutes. Remove from heat and set aside.

3. Whisk eggs, almond milk, and cinnamon in a large, flat-bottomed bowl.

4. Trim bread to fit bottom and sides of prepared ramekins. Dunk slices of bread in the egg wash as if making French toast. Line the bottom and sides of ramekins with the egg-soaked bread. Reserve two slices of bread for the top.

5. Spoon peach mixture into ramekins and top each with a slice of bread.

6. Bake for 35 minutes or until golden brown.

7. Serve warm or at room temperature.

▶ SERVES 2

Peach-Cinnamon Charlotte

1 teaspoon ghee or butter, plus more for greasing

1 teaspoon light olive oil

2 cups (fresh or frozen, thawed) diced peaches

¼ cup dried cranberries

¼ cup dry toasted walnuts

3 eggs

1 tablespoon almond milk (NS substitute rice milk)

½ teaspoon cinnamon (NS substitute ⅛ teaspoon nutmeg)

8 slices brown rice/millet bread

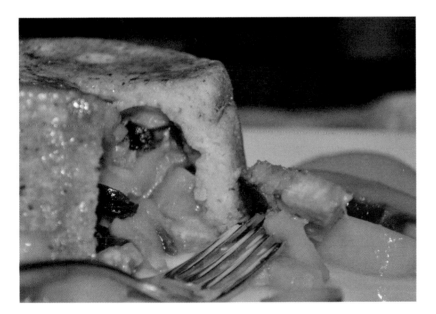

Type O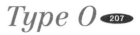

Carrot-Pineapple Cake with Chocolate-Chai Frosting

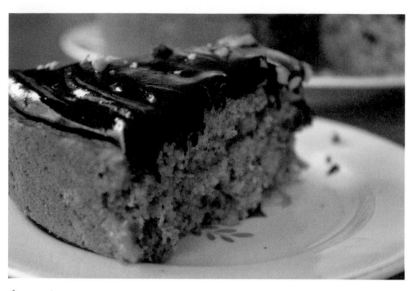

3 tablespoons butter or ghee, melted and cooled, plus more for greasing

1 cup shredded carrot

¾ cup diced pineapple

1 cup brown rice flour

1 cup millet flour

¼ cup arrowroot starch

3 teaspoons baking powder

1 teaspoon sea salt

½ teaspoon cinnamon (NS substitute ⅛ teaspoon nutmeg)

2 large egg yolks

1 cup finely chopped walnuts

½ cup agave

4 large egg whites

frosting:

½ cup almond milk (NS substitute rice milk)

4 tablespoons agave

1 teaspoon ground cinnamon (NS substitute ⅛ teaspoon nutmeg)

½ teaspoon ground ginger

⅛ teaspoon ground allspice

3 ounces 100 percent dark chocolate, grated

2 tablespoons ghee

2 tablespoons cocoa powder

¼ cup chopped walnuts, for garnish

1. Preheat oven to 350 degrees. Grease a 9-inch-round cake pan with butter and set aside.

2. Place shredded carrot and diced pineapple on a paper towel to absorb excess liquid, and set aside.

3. In a large bowl, combine flours, arrowroot starch, baking powder, salt, and cinnamon.

4. In a separate bowl, whisk together egg yolks, pineapple, carrots, walnuts, butter, and agave. Add to dry ingredients, stirring to combine, and set aside.

5. In a dry, glass bowl, beat egg whites until stiff peaks form. Fold egg whites into batter, one-third at a time. Pour into prepared cake pan.

6. Bake 35 to 40 minutes. Remove from oven, and cool for 5 minutes. Remove from pan onto a cooling rack to cool completely before frosting.

7. Combine almond milk and agave in a small saucepan with cinnamon, ginger, and allspice over medium heat, and heat 2 to 3 minutes, stirring occasionally. Place grated chocolate in a bowl with ghee. Pour hot milk mixture over chocolate, and whisk until smooth. Let cool completely. Add cocoa powder, and stir until mixture thickens.

8. Spread frosting on top of cooled cake, and sprinkle with walnuts. Serve same day for best results or store in a cool, dry place overnight or in the freezer for up to 1 month.

▶ SERVES 8

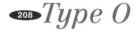

EAT RIGHT FOR YOUR TYPE PERSONALIZED COOKBOOK

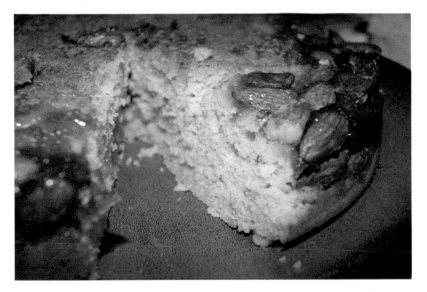

Upside-Down Almond Cake with Apricot Glaze

1. Preheat oven to 350 degrees. Grease a 9-inch-round cake pan, line with parchment paper, and set aside.

2. In a large bowl, whisk together flours, almond meal, baking powder, and salt. Set aside.

3. In a dry, glass bowl, beat egg whites with a hand mixer until stiff peaks form; set aside.

4. Mix remaining cake ingredients in a small bowl and add to dry mixture. Stir just until combined. Fold egg whites into batter, one-third at a time.

5. Scatter almonds evenly on the bottom of the cake pan. In a small saucepan, combine honey and apricot jam over low heat for 30 seconds, just until glaze thins out. Slowly pour over almonds in the bottom of the cake pan. Pour batter over almonds and bake for 40 minutes or until a cake tester comes out clean.

▶ SERVES 8

1 cup brown rice flour

½ cup millet flour

½ cup finely ground almond meal

2 teaspoons baking powder

½ teaspoon fine-grain sea salt

½ teaspoon lemon zest

4 large egg whites

2 large egg yolks

½ cup agave

2 tablespoons honey (NS substitute agave)

6 tablespoons ghee, softened

5 tablespoons almond milk (NS substitute rice milk)

topping:

1 cup whole almonds

2 tablespoons honey (NS substitute agave)

¼ cup sugar-free apricot jam (NS substitute cherry jam)

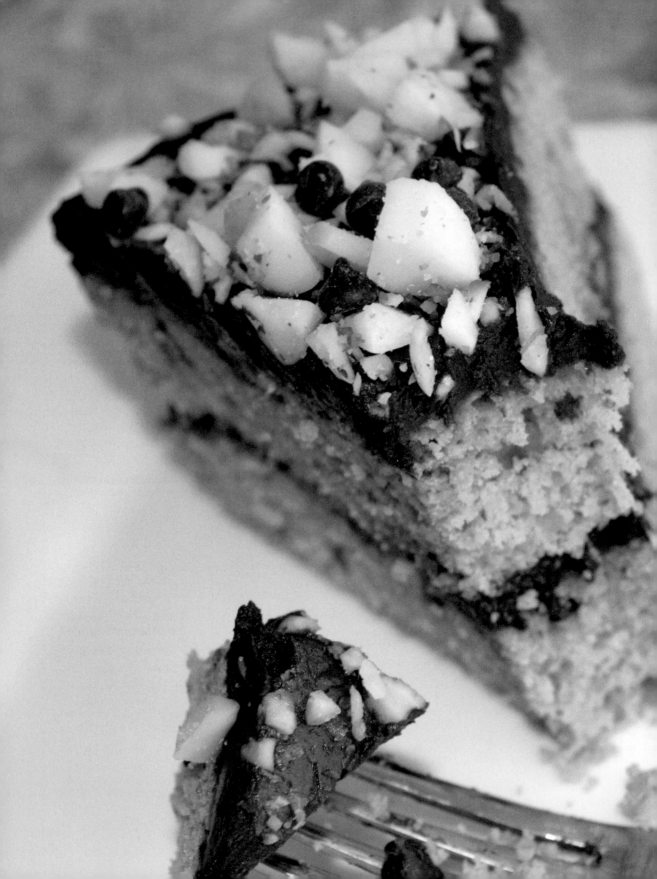

Matcha Cake with Chocolate Frosting

1. Preheat oven to 350 degrees. Grease two 9-inch-round cake pans with ghee, and set aside.

2. Combine matcha, flours, baking powder, salt, and cloves in a large bowl. Set aside.

3. In a separate bowl, whisk together lemon zest, agave, ghee, eggs, yolk, and almond milk, and set aside.

4. Place egg whites in a glass, copper, or metal bowl and beat on high until egg whites form stiff peaks.

5. Add wet mixture to dry mixture, and stir until well combined and free of lumps. Gently fold egg whites into batter, one-third at a time.

6. Divide batter evenly between prepared cake pans, bake on middle oven rack for 25 minutes, until cake is firm and cake tester comes out clean. Cool in cake pans for 10 minutes, then remove and cool fully on wire cooling racks.

7. Heat almond milk and agave in a small saucepan set over medium heat for 2 to 3 minutes. Place grated chocolate in a bowl with ghee. Pour hot milk mixture over chocolate and stir until smooth. Let cool completely. Add cocoa powder and stir until mixture thickens.

8. Spread slightly less than half the frosting on the first layer of cake, top with the second layer, and use an offset spatula to spread remaining frosting over the top of the second tier of cake. Sprinkle with toasted macadamia nuts and chocolate morsels.

▶ SERVES 8

4 tablespoons ghee or butter, melted and cooled, plus 1 tablespoon for greasing

1 tablespoon matcha powder

1½ cups brown rice flour

1 cup millet flour

3 teaspoons baking powder

½ teaspoon fine-grain sea salt

¼ teaspoon ground cloves

1 teaspoon lemon zest

½ cup agave

2 large eggs plus 1 egg yolk

⅓ cup almond milk (NS substitute rice milk)

3 large egg whites

frosting:

½ cup almond milk (NS substitute rice milk)

4 tablespoons agave

3 ounces 100 percent dark chocolate, grated

2 tablespoons ghee

2 tablespoons cocoa powder

⅔ cup chopped toasted macadamia nuts

¼ cup allergy-free chocolate morsels

 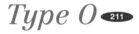

Crêpes with Raspberry Chutney (S)

¾ cup buckwheat flour (NS substitute rice flour)

¼ cup white rice flour or tapioca flour

1 tablespoon ghee plus 1 teaspoon, melted

½ teaspoon sea salt

2 large eggs

1½ cups almond milk (NS substitute rice milk)

raspberry chutney:

1 teaspoon ghee

1 Bosc pear, diced

1 teaspoon lemon zest

½ teaspoon grated fresh ginger

¼ cup sugar-free apricot jam (NS substitute cherry jam)

1 cup fresh, halved raspberries*

1. Whisk flours, 1 tablespoon ghee, salt, eggs, and milk in a large bowl. Cover and refrigerate for 1 hour.

2. While the batter chills, melt ghee in a medium skillet over medium heat and sauté pear for 3 to 4 minutes, until slightly browned and tender. Add lemon zest, ginger, and apricot jam to hot skillet, cooking for an additional 30 seconds. Remove from heat, and toss with fresh raspberries.

3. Heat a large, low-sided skillet over medium to medium-high heat, and (if not nonstick) brush with remaining melted ghee. Using a ¼-cup measure, spoon batter into the skillet and quickly turn in circular motions to spread batter into a very thin layer. Cook 1 minute, or until the edges start to pull away from pan and tiny bubbles appear in the center of the crepe. Using a large, flat spatula or carefully lifting edges with your hands, flip the crepe, and cook 1 minute on the other side. Repeat with remaining batter. Stack crepes on a plate, and keep warm until serving.

4. Serve warm with chutney and drizzled with Chocolate Syrup NS (page 219).

▶ SERVES 4

*Cranberries can be substituted here; add 1 tablespoon maple syrup.

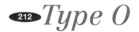

EAT RIGHT FOR YOUR TYPE PERSONALIZED COOKBOOK

featured ingredient

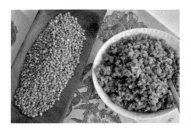

buckwheat

Buckwheat is a gluten-free, pyra-mid-shaped grain that has a slightly sweet, nutty flavor and is high in protein. It is a delicious al-ternative to wheat, and pairs per-fectly with fresh fruit and chocolate! Buckwheat can also be eaten as a whole-grain side to any meal, much like rice and quinoa. It is quick to cook and a nutritious variation on your weeknight meal.

Banana-Based Ice Cream: 4 Ways

basic recipe:

4 semi-ripened bananas, unpeeled

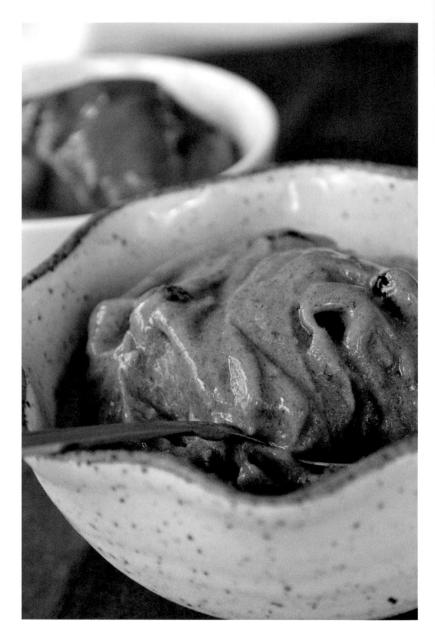

1. Freeze bananas overnight. Once frozen, peel and slice. Add to food processor and blend about 2 minutes until bananas resemble creamy ice cream. Spoon into a bowl and serve. Add the following combinations for variety.

option 1: double chocolate

1 tablespoon cocoa powder
1 tablespoon agave
¼ cup mini dark chocolate chips

1. Add cocoa powder and agave to frozen bananas in the food processor and blend until smooth and creamy. Fold in chocolate chips and serve.

option 2: maple pecan/agave pecan

⅓ cup pecans, chopped
2 tablespoons maple syrup, divided (NS substitute agave)
⅛ teaspoon salt

1. Toast pecans in a small skillet over medium heat. Add 1 tablespoon maple syrup and salt, and set aside to cool.

2. Add remaining maple syrup to food processor with frozen bananas and blend until smooth and creamy. Fold in cooled pecans and serve.

option 3: blueberry proberry™

1 teaspoon Proberry 3™ Liquid*
1 tablespoon agave
½ cup (fresh or frozen) blueberries

1. Add Proberry 3™ Liquid and agave to bananas in food processor and blend until smooth and creamy. Stir in blueberries and serve.

▶ SERVES 4

*Information about purchasing Proberry 3™ Liquid can be found in Appendix II: Products (page 250).

tip: If bananas become too soft while adding other ingredients, simply store in a glass container and freeze for an additional 2 hours. Ice cream stays fresh in freezer for up to 1 week.

Ginger-Rice Pudding

1 cup long-grain, brown basmati rice

½ teaspoon sea salt

3½ cups almond milk, divided (NS substitute rice milk)

1 tablespoon fresh ginger, peeled and grated

⅛ teaspoon ground cardamom (optional)

½ teaspoon ground cinnamon (NS omit cinnamon and add ⅛ teaspoon nutmeg)

2 large egg yolks

2 tablespoons brown rice flour

1 tablespoon blackstrap molasses

1 tablespoon maple syrup

½ cup diced, dried mango

1. In a medium saucepan, combine rice, salt, and 2 cups almond milk. Bring to a boil, cover, reduce heat, and simmer 45 to 50 minutes, until rice has absorbed all the liquid in the pan.

2. In a small saucepan, combine remaining 1½ cups milk, ginger, cardamom, and cinnamon over medium heat until warm, about 4 to 6 minutes. In a small bowl, whisk together egg yolks, flour, molasses, and maple syrup. Temper the egg mixture by slowly adding a ladle of the warm milk to the eggs, whisking continuously. Add egg mixture to milk mixture, and whisk over medium heat until the mixture is thick and resembles the consistency of yogurt, 4 to 5 minutes. Remove from heat.

3. Add mango and milk mixture to rice. Cook an additional 3 to 5 minutes over low heat, stirring continuously, until pudding is thick and creamy.

4. Serve warm.

▶ SERVES 6

EAT RIGHT FOR YOUR TYPE PERSONALIZED COOKBOOK

Stocks, Condiments, and Sauces

Ketchup Substitute ■ *Herb Dressing* NS ■ *Carrot-Ginger Dressing* NS ■ *Chocolate Syrup* NS ■ *Cinnamon Syrup* ■ *Chicken or Turkey Stock* NS ■ *Beef Stock* NS ■ *Vegetable Stock* NS ■ *Basic Gluten-Free Bread Crumbs* NS

Ketchup Substitute

1 teaspoon olive oil

2 tablespoons finely chopped onion

½ cup organic tomato paste

1 tablespoon agave

2 tablespoons apple juice (NS substitute pear juice)

½ teaspoon sea salt

¼ teaspoon black pepper

1 tablespoon lemon juice

1 teaspoon blackstrap molasses

1. Heat olive oil in a small skillet over medium heat, and sauté onion for 3 to 4 minutes. Add remaining ingredients and simmer about 4 minutes. Spoon into a bowl or glass jar and let cool. Store in the refrigerator and use as ketchup substitute.

Herb Dressing NS

¼ cup finely chopped fresh basil

2 tablespoons finely chopped fresh parsley

2 tablespoons finely chopped fresh chives

2 small cloves garlic, minced

½ cup extra virgin olive oil

⅔ cup lemon juice

½ teaspoon crushed red pepper

Sea salt, to taste

1. Whisk herbs, garlic, oil, lemon juice, and crushed red pepper together in a small bowl, or pour ingredients in a glass jar with a sealable lid and shake vigorously to combine. Season with sea salt, to taste.

2. Store salad dressing in a glass jar or dispenser in the refrigerator for up to 1 week. Recipe can also be doubled.

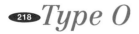

Carrot-Ginger Dressing NS

1. Place carrots, olive oil, ginger, and lemon juice in a food processor and pulse until a smooth consistency is reached. If the mixture is too thick, add water 1 tablespoon at a time.

2. Season with sea salt, to taste, and store in a glass container or dispenser in the refrigerator for up to 1 week.

2 medium carrots, chopped

1 tablespoon olive oil

1 (1-inch) piece fresh ginger, peeled

1 tablespoon fresh lemon juice

Sea salt, to taste

Chocolate Syrup NS

1. Whisk agave and cocoa powder vigorously in a bowl to incorporate. Store in a clean, glass dispenser or a glass container, and drizzle over pancakes or fruit, or add to smoothies for a special treat.

2. Store in a cool, dry place for up to 2 weeks.

1 cup agave

2 tablespoons cocoa powder

 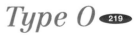

Cinnamon Syrup

2 teaspoons butter

1 cup agave

2 teaspoons cinnamon

1. Melt butter in a saucepan over medium-low heat. Add agave and cinnamon, whisking until smooth and combined. Remove from heat and let cool completely.

2. Store in the refrigerator in a clean, glass dispenser or container for up to 2 weeks.

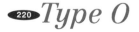

Chicken or Turkey Stock NS

1. Bring all ingredients to a gentle boil in a large stockpot. As the stock boils, use a large spoon to skim foam and impurities off the top and discard. When the stock comes to a full boil, reduce heat, cover and simmer 3 hours.

2. Remove ingredients from stock and strain into a clean bowl or pot. Let cool (not more than 4 hours), then package and refrigerate.

3. Store in glass containers in the refrigerator for up to 3 days or in the freezer for 2 months.

4 pounds chicken or turkey thighs and breast

3 large carrots, peeled and diced

1 celery root, peeled and diced

2 cloves garlic, peeled

1 Vidalia onion, chopped

4 quarts water

2 teaspoons sea salt

3 sprigs fresh thyme

3 sprigs fresh rosemary

5 sprigs parsley

2 bay leaves

 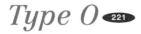

Beef Stock (NS)

3 bay leaves

4 sprigs fresh thyme

4 pounds beef bones

2 teaspoons olive oil

Sea salt, to taste

2 Vidalia onions, rough chopped

4 carrots, rough chopped

1 cup parsnips, rough chopped

4 quarts water, divided

2 cloves garlic, peeled

1 cup red wine

½ cup tomato paste

1. Preheat oven to 450 degrees.

2. Gather bay leaves and thyme, and tie with kitchen twine to secure together or wrap in cheesecloth, and set aside.

3. Place beef bones in a baking dish and brush with olive oil and a dash of sea salt. Roast for 30 minutes. Turn beef and add onion, carrots, and parsnips to the roasting pan, and bake for 30 minutes. Remove from oven and place beef bones and vegetables into a stockpot.

4. Deglaze baking dish with 2 cups of water, scraping up the bits off the bottom. If it is difficult to deglaze, simply place the baking dish over the burners on the stove over medium-low heat and continue scraping until all bits come up.

5. Pour mixture into the stockpot and add water, herbs, garlic, red wine, and tomato paste. Simmer 3 to 4 hours, skimming the top of the stock with a spoon to remove impurities while it cooks.

6. Strain stock into a clean pot and cool completely. Store in the refrigerator for 2 days or in the freezer for 2 months.

Vegetable Stock NS

1. Heat olive oil in a large stockpot over medium heat, and sauté onion, celery root, parsnip, carrots, and fennel for 8 to 10 minutes, just until tender. Add water and remaining ingredients and bring to a boil.

2. Cover, reduce heat to low, and cook 30 minutes. (Vegetable stock has a quick cooking time because vegetables give up their flavor quickly, as opposed to meats and bones.)

3. Strain stock into a clean pot, cool, and store in the refrigerator for 3 to 5 days or in the freezer for 2 to 3 months.

2 teaspoons olive oil

2 onions, chopped

1 celery root, peeled and chopped

3 large parsnips, peeled and chopped

3 large carrots, peeled and chopped

2 bulbs fennel, chopped

4 quarts water

3 tomatoes, halved

3 bay leaves

1 clove garlic, peeled

5 sprigs parsley

5 sprigs thyme

2 teaspoons sea salt

Basic Gluten-Free Bread Crumbs NS

4 slices gluten-free bread

1. Toast bread and let cool. Pulse in a food processor until coarse crumbs form.

2. For flavored bread crumbs, add dried herbs and seasonings such as parsley, rosemary, thyme, sage, and/or basil, onion or garlic powder, and salt.

Useful Tools

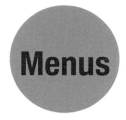
Menus

Substitutions

An integral part of acclimating to your new diet is being able to fill the void left by your *Best Avoided* list. Below is a list of substitutions to help you along the way. A number of these are not direct substitutions, but you will see from recipes in this book how they are adapted to work in place of items on your *Best Avoided* list.

BREAD—If you cannot have spelt, there are several breads containing brown rice and millet. Though not sold in many stores, most are accessible online. They are often less expensive to order online in bulk and store in the freezer. Bakers make varieties with flax, garlic, basil, cinnamon, and banana walnut, as well as bagels, rolls, hot dog buns, and even flatbreads, which are a perfect base for pizza. If you are able to eat spelt, there are more options available. Just be sure to read labels carefully because many breads contain ingredients that may not work for your blood type. In addition, because grains in general are not as *Beneficial* to Type Os, another option is to swap bread for lettuces like Boston Bibb or endive to make little pockets for sandwich fillings.

PASTA—Wheat- and gluten-free pasta is fairly easy to come by these days, and found in most grocery stores. You want to look for a brand with ingredients containing no more than brown rice flour (or bran) and water. When cooking gluten-free, it is important to know that, if boiled too long, the noodles will become undesirably mushy and fall apart. You should cook pasta 3 to 4 minutes short of the recommended package cooking time to ensure a good, slightly al dente texture.

BUTTER—Most Type Os are allowed butter and in some cases, it is a *Beneficial* food. If you are unable to have butter, however, the best alternative is ghee, which is simply clarified butter. When butter is heated, it separates and the lactose comes to the top and the fat remains on the bottom. When the lactose is removed, what remains is called ghee. Use it just like butter, to spread on toast or add to rice or vegetables.

OIL—Coconut and soy oils are not recommended for most Type O diets. Olive oil is a *Beneficial* food for all Os, and is a great alternative for cooking and baking. Use light olive oil for baking to avoid a pervasive olive taste in your baked goods. Extra virgin olive oil is terrific for dressing salads or even a medium-heat stir-fry.

SUGAR—There are a few alternatives to raw sugar, however, they are mostly liquid, so swapping 1:1 is not the best strategy. For Type Os, the best alternatives to sugar are blackstrap molasses, agave, maple syrup, maple sugar, and honey. Most of the recipes in this book call for agave and molasses because they are the most universally *Beneficial* sweeteners for the Blood Type Diet. You can, however, experiment with swapping agave or molasses for a combination of other sweeteners.

FLOUR—The best flours for wheat- and gluten-free baking come from using a combination for texture and taste. Recipes in this book use combinations such as brown rice flour, tapioca, and millet. Tapioca can also be swapped out for any acceptable fine, starchy flour such as arrowroot starch. Brown rice flour can be swapped out for another hearty grain such as millet, buckwheat, amaranth, or quinoa. Using a combination helps to significantly improve texture, taste, and quality of gluten-free baking.

Non-Secretor Substitutions

Non-Secretors have to avoid a few staples that Secretors are allowed; these are listed in each recipe, but a few basics are included below. Substitute any recipe containing almond milk with rice milk; butter with ghee; tapioca flour with arrowroot starch or white rice flour; and omit cinnamon or follow specific recipe directions for a replacement.

A great everyday baking mix for Type O is:
    2 parts brown rice flour (⅔ cup for one batch)

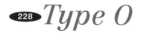
Type O

EAT RIGHT FOR YOUR TYPE PERSONALIZED COOKBOOK

1 part millet or teff flour (⅓ cup for one batch)

1 part arrowroot starch or tapioca flour (⅓ cup for one batch)

Add 2 teaspoons baking powder and ½ teaspoon sea salt to
each batch.

Menu Planning

The following are suggestions to show you how to put the recipes in this book together to create weekly menus for you and your family. They are arranged in a way to keep a balanced diet, but feel free to mix and match as you see fit. If you plan to follow the menu exactly, read it thoroughly ahead of time so you can see where you would need to buy a little extra to account for leftovers, and where it would be practical to plan/prep ahead. The purpose of menu planning is to make life as easy as possible by utilizing leftovers and planning more involved meals for weekends.

In addition to the list below, make sure you are drinking a minimum of 6 (8-oz.) glasses of water per day to stay properly hydrated.

MENU PLANNING TIPS:

■ If you are working full-time or have difficulty preparing meals during the week, use time on the weekend to prepare snacks and a few meals for the week by pre-washing vegetables and lettuce. This will significantly cut down on weekday duties. A few foods that stay well and you should always have on hand are: Flax Crackers, Blackstrap-Cherry Granola, Spicy Rosemary-Nut Clusters, and occasionally a Unibar® Protein Bar.

■ If you don't like leftovers, it's time to start liking them! Honestly, leftovers are the most delightful time-savers you could imagine. Pair them with a fresh salad or toss in a soup, and they will become your best friend, too.

■ When making something like bruschetta, double the topping recipe and store in a sealable glass container in the refrigerator for up to 1 week. That way you make it once and use as many times as you want it.

■ When baking breads, muffins, or even sweet treats, freeze leftovers in sealable glass containers to keep them fresh. If, for example, you have Pumpkin Muffins in the freezer, you can pop them in the oven or toaster oven at 200 degrees for 10 to 15 minutes and they will be perfectly toasty and ready to eat. Frozen chocolate chip cookies are also delicious and don't require defrosting—one of the magical things about gluten-free flour.

Four-Week Meal Planner

Week 1

Sunday

BREAKFAST: Wild-Rice Waffles with sliced banana and raw walnuts

LUNCH: Ratatouille NS

SNACK: Celery Sticks with Curried Egg Salad NS

DINNER: Beef Tips with Wild Mushrooms NS

Monday

BREAKFAST: Granola–Nut Butter Fruit Slices, rice cereal, and almond milk with fresh blueberries and green tea

LUNCH: Leftover Beef Tips with Wild Mushrooms NS with mixed green salad dressed with lemon and olive oil

SNACK: Pear and Apple Chips and Spicy Rosemary-Nut Mix

DINNER: Lemon-Ginger Salmon with Brown Rice Salad NS

Tuesday

BREAKFAST: Scrambled Eggs with Blueberry-Macadamia Muffins and green tea

LUNCH: Raw Kale Salad with Zesty Lime Dressing NS and leftover Lemon-Ginger Salmon

SNACK: Flax Crackers NS and Heirloom Tomato Salsa

DINNER: Crispy-Coated Turkey Tenderloins with Apricot Dipping Sauce and Tomato and Broccoli Ragu NS

Wednesday

BREAKFAST: Homemade Turkey Breakfast Sausage with sliced mango and green tea

LUNCH: Raw Kale Salad with Zesty Lime Dressing NS and leftover Crispy-Coated Turkey Tenderloins with Apricot Dipping Sauce

SNACK: Pear and Apple Chips and Spicy Rosemary-Nut Mix

DINNER: Grilled Radicchio and Walnut-Spinach Pesto NS

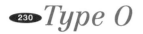

Thursday

BREAKFAST: Blueberry-Macadamia Muffins with leftover Home-made Turkey Breakfast Sausage and green tea

LUNCH: Greens and Beans Salad NS with rotisserie chicken

SNACK: Protein Blend™ Powder—Type O drink

DINNER: Tangy Pineapple and Beef Kabobs NS with Autumn Roasted Roots NS

Friday

BREAKFAST: Quinoa Muesli, banana slices, blueberries, and green tea

LUNCH: Leftover Greens and Beans Salad NS with leftover Tangy Pineapple and Beef Kabobs NS

SNACK: Carob–Walnut Butter–Stuffed Figs NS

DINNER: Roasted Tomato and Broccoli Mac and Cheese and Garlic-Creamed Spinach

Saturday

BREAKFAST: Broccoli-Feta Frittata with pineapple and green tea

LUNCH: ½ Bacon Grilled Cheese with Tomato-Basil Soup NS

SNACK: Almond Butter Rice Cakes with Mini Chips

DINNER: Seafood Paella

Week 2

Sunday

BREAKFAST: Cherry Scones with almond butter and green tea

LUNCH: White Bean Stew NS

SNACK: Grilled Pineapple with Cinnamon Syrup

DINNER: Moroccan Lamb Tagine

Monday

BREAKFAST: Breakfast Egg Salad

LUNCH: Mint and Cherry Tomato Tabbouleh NS with leftover Moroccan Lamb Tagine

SNACK: Homemade Applesauce

DINNER: Shredded Turkey Bake

Tuesday

BREAKFAST: Quinoa Muesli with sliced bananas and fresh blueberries

 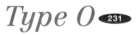

LUNCH: Leftover Shredded Turkey Bake with mixed greens dressed in olive oil and lemon

SNACK: Grilled Pineapple with Cinnamon Syrup

DINNER: Beef and Shredded Escarole Soup NS and Red Quinoa–Mushroom Casserole with Fried Eggs NS

Wednesday

BREAKFAST: Swiss Chard and Cremini Frittata NS with mango slices and green tea

LUNCH: Leftover Red Quinoa–Mushroom Casserole with Fried Eggs NS

SNACK: Toasty Pizza Bites

DINNER: Parchment-Baked Snapper NS

Thursday

BREAKFAST: Broccoli-Feta Frittata with green tea

LUNCH: Adzuki Hummus Sandwich NS

SNACK: Homemade Applesauce

DINNER: Meat Loaf with Spicy Collards NS and Baked Beans NS

Friday

BREAKFAST: Granola–Nut Butter Fruit Slices with green tea

LUNCH: Leftover Meat Loaf sandwiches

SNACK: Protein Blend™ Powder—Type O drink

DINNER: Spicy Seafood Stew NS

Saturday

BREAKFAST: Brown Rice Pancakes with scrambled eggs and green tea

LUNCH: Salmon-Salad Radicchio Cups

SNACK: Crispy Spring Vegetable Cakes NS

DINNER: Sweet Potato Gnocchi with Basil-Cranberry Sauce NS with grilled chicken

Week 3

Sunday

BREAKFAST: Pear-Rosemary Bread NS with poached egg and green tea

LUNCH: Philly Cheesesteak Sandwich

SNACK: Crudités and Creamy Goat Cheese Dip S (S Only!)

DINNER: Turkey Mole Drumsticks with Whipped Sweet Potato Soufflé and Sweet and Crunchy Kohlrabi Slaw NS

Monday

BREAKFAST: Creamy Banana–Nut Butter Smoothie and green tea

LUNCH: Leftover Turkey Mole Drumsticks and Sweet and Crunchy Kohlrabi Slaw NS

SNACK: Unibar® Protein Bar

DINNER: Salmon–Black Bean Cakes with Creamy Cilantro Sauce NS and Roasted Wakame and Fennel Salad NS

Tuesday

BREAKFAST: Pear-Rosemary Bread NS with scrambled eggs and green tea

LUNCH: Leftover Salmon–Black Bean Cakes with Creamy Cilantro Sauce with leftover Roasted Wakame and Fennel Salad NS dressed in lemon and olive oil

SNACK: Marinated Mozzarella S (S Only!) with Flax Crackers NS

DINNER: Hearty Slow-Cooker Turkey Stew NS with Sweet-and-Salty Brussels

Wednesday

BREAKFAST: Turkey Bacon–Spinach Squares and green tea

LUNCH: Leftover Hearty Slow-Cooker Turkey Stew NS

SNACK: Unibar® Protein Bar

DINNER: Broccoli–Northern Bean Soup NS with Green Tea–Poached Chicken NS

Thursday

BREAKFAST: Blackstrap-Cherry Granola NS, rice cereal, and almond milk with fresh blueberries and green tea

LUNCH: Shredded leftover Green Tea–Poached Chicken NS with cranberries and walnuts over spinach greens with olive oil and lemon

SNACK: Marinated Mozzarella (S Only!) with Flax Crackers NS

DINNER: Fig-Stuffed Turkey Breasts NS with Roasted Pumpkin with Fried Sage NS

Friday

BREAKFAST: Homemade Turkey Breakfast Sausage with sliced mango and green tea

 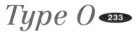

LUNCH: Leftover Fig-Stuffed Turkey Breasts NS over Raw Kale Salad with Zesty Lime Dressing NS

SNACK: Unibar® Protein Bar

DINNER: Beef Tips with Wild Mushrooms NS with Roasted Parsnip Soup

Saturday

BREAKFAST: Spinach-Zucchini Soufflé and green tea

LUNCH: Crunchy Kohlrabi Spring Rolls with Sweet Cherry Dip NS

SNACK: Farmer Cheese and Beet-Endive Cups

DINNER: Spring Pesto Pasta with grilled chicken

Week 4

Sunday

BREAKFAST: Savory Herb and Cheese Bread Pudding

LUNCH: Adzuki Hummus Sandwich NS

SNACK: Fruit Salad with Mint-Lime Dressing NS

DINNER: Sweet Potato Shepherd's Pie with Roasted Escarole NS

Monday

BREAKFAST: Maple-Sausage Scramble and green tea

LUNCH: Leftover Sweet Potato Shepherd's Pie

SNACK: Artichoke Bruschetta

DINNER: Baked Mahimahi with Crunchy Fennel Salad and Herbed Quinoa

Tuesday

BREAKFAST: Pumpkin Muffins with Carob Drizzle with almond butter and green tea

LUNCH: Baked Falafel NS and Roasted Tomato Greek Salad

SNACK: Fruit Salad with Mint-Lime Dressing NS

DINNER: Sun-Dried Tomato Burgers on Millet Buns and Crispy Walnut Bacon–Wrapped Asparagus NS

Wednesday

BREAKFAST: Granola–Nut Butter Fruit Slices with Mango-Kale Smoothie and green tea

LUNCH: Rotisserie chicken with leftover Crispy Walnut Bacon–Wrapped Asparagus NS wrapped in Boston Bibb lettuce cups

SNACK: Crudités and Creamy Goat Cheese Dip s (S Only!)

DINNER: Turkey-Ginger Stir-Fry NS with Carrot-Ginger Soup NS

Thursday

BREAKFAST: Breakfast Egg Salad with green tea

LUNCH: Leftover Carrot-Ginger Soup NS and ½ Adzuki Hummus Sandwich NS

SNACK: Artichoke Bruschetta

DINNER: Pasta Carbonara with Crispy Kale with Greens and Beans Salad NS

Friday

BREAKFAST: Pumpkin Muffins with Carob Drizzle with almond butter and green tea

LUNCH: Leftover Greens and Beans Salad NS with walnuts and fresh mozzarella cheese

SNACK: Crudités and Creamy Goat Cheese Dip s (S Only!)

DINNER: Fish Tacos with Sweet Mango-Bean Salad

Saturday

BREAKFAST: Cinnamon-Millet Crêpes and green tea

LUNCH: Melted Mozzarella–Onion Soup

SNACK: Baked Grapefruit with Honey and Cinnamon

DINNER: Chicken Pot Pie with Crunchy Topping NS

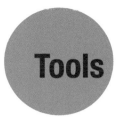

Tools

YOU CAN FIND helpful tools on our website at www.4yourtype .com/cookbooks.asp. From there, you can download the following PDFs and print them from your computer.

- Food Journal
   Keep track of every meal with this handy log.

- Tracking Your Progress
   This is an additional log to help you focus on your goals.

- Shopping List
   Make your shopping trip easy with this list of *Beneficial* foods for your type.

TYPE O SHOPPING LIST:
Produce:

Artichokes	Figs	Spinach
Bananas	Kale	Sweet potatoes
Blueberries	Lettuce	Watermelon
Broccoli	Mango	
Cherries	Onions	

Baking:

Agave	Millet flour
Arrowroot starch	Sea salt
Baking powder	
Brown rice flour	
(*Neutral*)	

Dairy:

Butter

Eggs

Feta cheese

Mozzarella cheese

Meat/Seafood:

Beef	Halibut	Red snapper
Cod	Lamb	Turkey

Miscellaneous:

Adzuki beans	Carob	Olive oil
Almond butter	Cayenne pepper	Parsley
Almonds	Curry powder	Seltzer
Black-eyed peas	Flaxseed	Walnuts
Brown rice bread	Ginger tea	
(Neutral)	Green tea	

Please note: this shopping list only highlights the most frequently used *Beneficial* and some *Neutral* foods for Type O. For a complete list of *Beneficial*, *Neutral*, and *Avoids*, you should refer to *Eat Right 4 Your Type*, *Live Right 4 Your Type*, or *Blood Type O Food, Beverage, and Supplement Lists* or your SWAMI personalized nutrition plan.

Time to Think Green

MICHEL NISCHAN IS a sustainable chef, cookbook author, and connoisseur of local, healthy food. He wrote in one of his books, *Sustainably Delicious: Making the World a Better Place, One Recipe at a Time*, "Where there is flavor, there are nutrients, and where there are nutrients, there is health." It is well known by chefs around the globe that the best food comes from the freshest ingredients and nothing is fresher than a tomato grown in your own backyard or at the local farm. When you meander through your local farmers market and browse fruits and vegetables picked at their peak of freshness, the smells, touch, and tastes become infinitely more vibrant than a similar stroll through the supermarket. If you start any meal with fresh, local, whole-food ingredients, almost anything you make will be the best-tasting food, and the best for your health.

Here are a few highlights on buying organic, avoiding toxins in your kitchen, and shopping for the freshest fruits and vegetables.

Quick Review of the Terms

Whenever possible, buy organic food and grass-fed beef. Why? Conventional fruits and vegetables are sprayed with harmful chemicals such as herbicides, pesticides, and insecticides. The chemicals used in these substances can disrupt hormones, and potentially cause cancer, allergies, asthma, and other health issues. Conventionally raised meat, dairy, and poultry exist in poor conditions and are fed for the purpose of fast weight gain, which is taxing to their health. As a result, animals are given antibiotics, which end up in the meat you buy at the grocery store. In addition, some animals are put on hormones to bulk up their bodies, making their meat artificially larger and, therefore, more desirable to consumers' eyes. Eating meat is a terrific source of healing food for Type Os, but if the meat is contaminated with hormones and antibiotics and causing unnecessary disruptions to your system, the goodness is essentially negated.

Here are a few definitions to sort out some of the confusion:

100 Percent USDA Certified Organic—This means that the product you purchase must contain only organic ingredients, minus water and salt. Knowing the abbreviation USDA is an easy way to identify foods that are 100 percent certified organic.

Organic—Products must contain a minimum of 95 percent organic ingredients. Each ingredient within the product that is organic must also be labeled as such.

Made with Organic Ingredients—This label indicates that 70 percent or more ingredients contained in the product are organic. The word *organic* cannot be prominently displayed on the product.

Natural—The product contains no artificial ingredients or added color and is processed in a way that does not fundamentally alter its ingredients.

No Hormones—This term can only be used for beef. Poultry and pork are not allowed to be raised using hormones so the label is unnecessary.

Grass-Fed—This term applies to animals that are solely fed grass and hay.

Free-Range—This indicates that animals are allowed access to the outside. This label is tricky, however, because there are a large number of farms that keep their animals in poor conditions but allow a tiny space for "outdoor access" in order to be labeled "Free Range." To determine if the eggs you buy are coming from humane farms, check out http://www.cornucopia.org/organic-egg-scorecard for a scored list.

Tips for Buying Local and Organic
Choosing Food That Is in Season

The phrase *in season* is tossed around a lot, but what is the benefit of eating in season? Taste. Obviously, it also has a significant environmental impact, but the difference between eating a fresh-off-the-vine heirloom tomato versus a genetically modified tomato from the grocery store is striking enough to convince even the harshest of skeptics. Eating in season also ensures that you are rotating the kinds of vegetables in your diet, and, as a result, the nutrients. There is nothing more refreshing than fresh watermelon in the summer or roasted pumpkin in the fall. Make a habit of eating only the best by choosing local, organic food that is in season.

Where to Find Fresh Food in Season?

Look for local listings indicating farm stands or farmers markets. Most farms are also happy to show you around if you want to stop by for a visit or take your children to see how food is grown and raised. A terrific resource for finding local food is www.localharvest.org. Just fill out your city/state and you will be provided with a listing of local and organic food happenings. Eating in season is more satisfying to the body and palate.

Local or Organic?

Sometimes we have to make the choice between eating local food or organically grown food, and it can be confusing. Local food is terrific because of its freshness and limited impact on the environment; it does not have to be shipped all the way from Chile to get to your table. Food that is organic, however, is grown without harmful chemicals that are detrimental to your health but that also negatively impact our environment. I typically reach for the organic if I cannot have both. In an ideal world we wouldn't have to choose between organic and pesticide-free foods, but sometimes that is the choice we are faced with as customers. Thankfully, many independent, local farms practice organic farming, which can limit the need for these choices.

Healthy Choices on a Budget?

At some point, we all have to watch what we spend on everything, including food. The number-one tip for maintaining a healthy diet on a budget is prioritizing. If you are eating right for your blood type, you will be cutting out extras like potato chips, soda, prepared dips, cookies, and most overly processed foods. This alone will start to make room in your budget for healthier alternatives. Additionally, buying food in season is far less expensive than buying those same foods out of season. For example, a pint of organic blueberries in the middle of the winter can cost up to $6.99; the same pint at the farmers market in the summer can go as low as $2.99. When stocking up on grains or nuts, be savvy and buy in bulk. Nuts contain fats that if left in your pantry could spoil quickly, however, so store excess nuts in the freezer and they'll keep for several months. Buying in bulk also means you are cutting down on the cost and waste of excess packaging, which you definitely pay for.

Finally, prioritizing your organic purchases will save you a bundle. There are twelve fruits and vegetables that carry the most pesticide residue; therefore, buying these ingredients organic should take priority. (See the foods on the Dirty Dozen, listed below.) If you are on a budget, don't cut out these foods entirely, simply cut back how many you buy in one trip. Try to pick one or two ingredients that you must buy organic and supplement them with produce known to carry the lowest levels of pesticides, also known as the Clean Fifteen.

Dirty Dozen/Clean Fifteen

Below is a list of the Dirty Dozen*. Try to buy these organic as often as possible to reduce your exposure to pesticides.

1. Apples
2. Celery
3. Strawberries (*Avoid* for Type O Non-Secretors)
4. Peaches
5. Spinach
6. Nectarines (imported)
7. Grapes (imported)
8. Sweet bell peppers
9. Potatoes (*Avoid* for O)
10. Blueberries (domestic)
11. Lettuce
12. Kale/collard greens

Listed here is the Clean Fifteen*, a list of produce that has the smallest traces of pesticides and are therefore safest to buy in their conventional form. If it is possible, however, choosing organic is always better for yourself and the environment.

1. Onions
2. Sweet corn (*Avoid* for O)
3. Pineapples
4. Avocados (*Avoid* for O)
5. Asparagus
6. Sweet peas
7. Mangoes
8. Eggplant
9. Cantaloupe (domestic) (*Avoid* for O)
10. Kiwis (*Avoid* for O)
11. Cabbage (*Avoid* for O)
12. Watermelon
13. Sweet potatoes
14. Grapefruit
15. Mushrooms

*Dirty Dozen and Clean Fifteen taken from the Environmental Working Group website, www.ewg.org.

Safe Food Storage

The first question is what is safe? As most of us are aware, there is a chemical in most plastics called Biphenol-A (BPA), which, when ingested, acts as a hormone disrupter. Recently conducted studies reported that BPA negatively affects hormone levels, which can lead to obesity, as well as problems with thyroid function, and the risk of certain cancers.

Where Is BPA Found?

BPA is a compound found in consumer products such as plastic containers, water bottles, plastic wrap, cans, and some cartons. Plastics labeled 3, 6, or 7 for recycling purposes often contain BPA.

What Makes BPA Leach into Our Food?

Cans contain BPA in their lining. Therefore, when a can contains foods with high levels of acidity (like tomatoes), there is a greater likelihood that BPA will seep into the food it contains. Foods with high acidity also affect plastics, but a drastic change in the temperature of plastics (like freezing or being left in a warm car) will have the same leaching effect.

How Do I Avoid It?

Thankfully, it is getting easier and easier to avoid BPAs, mostly because they are being banned by the government in most products for children. Additionally, the more we know about the harmful effects of BPA, the more demand there is in the market for products that are free of this harm-

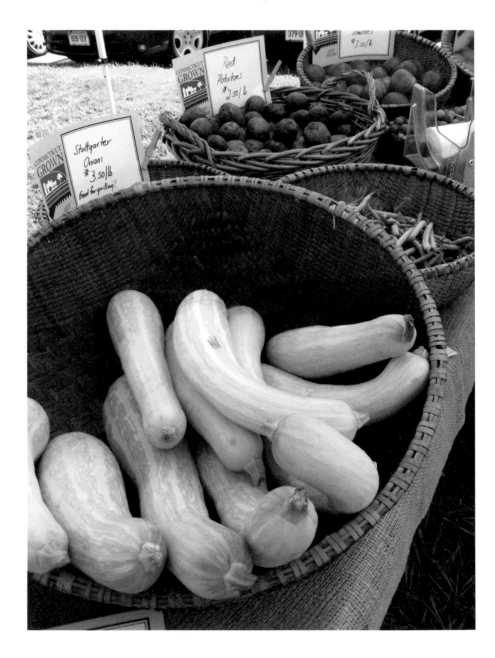

ful chemical. There are many companies now offering BPA-free products. A terrific alternative to canned tomatoes are products packaged by Tetra Pak; all of its packaging is BPA-free. Additionally, look for foods packaged in glass jars as opposed to cans or plastics.

What Should Be Done About Buying Food in Plastic/Cans?

The best way to purchase food is fresh, in glass, or in Tetra Pak cartons. Meats and seafood that are packaged in plastic by your butcher can be swapped out at home for further storage. If you feel inclined, however, let your butcher know you would prefer your food wrapped in paper. If enough people speak up, a change will certainly happen.

How Do I Pack Safe School Lunches?

Traditionally, kids' lunch boxes and plastic bottles contain BPAs. The good news is that there are an increasing number of BPA-free options now available; you just have to look for them. Due to recent studies about the adverse effects of BPA on health, most companies are trying to or are required by law to switch to BPA-free packaging. That being said, glass containers with sealable lids are available in many different sizes and are another great alternative to plastic.

NOTE: Get kids involved, so they start learning young. Let them help you in the process of preparing and packing their lunches. This allows them to learn about healthier nutrition. Choose fun, nontoxic snack packs for them to store their lunches.

Cleaning up the Kitchen

What's Wrong with Chemicals?

Traditional household cleaners contain chemicals such as alkylphenols, alkylphenol ethoxylates, ammonia, chlorine, and diethanolamine, just to name a few. These chemicals can cause allergies, skin irritation, asthma, and potentially much more serious health problems. Avoiding these chemicals and others in our environment is pretty much impossible, but what we can do is become aware of where they exist, and limit our exposure as much as possible. The first step is cleaning out your detergents, bleach, disinfectant sprays, or wipes along with any other cleaning products.

Is It More Expensive to Use Natural Cleaners?

If you're smart about it, it doesn't have to be. In fact, cleaning with natural products can actually be less expensive. For example, vinegar is mentioned below as a replacement to some cleaning products. A generic brand of vinegar is about $0.02/ounce, and a little definitely goes a long way.

What Are Some Household Products That Can Clean Well?

The best nontoxic cleaners are vinegar, baking soda, lemon juice, and club soda. Vinegar is a natural disinfectant, and believe it or not, deodorizer. You can use it on floors, countertops, sinks, and any surface that needs cleaning. Baking soda mixed with water is slightly abrasive and can be used to clean stainless steel and carpets, and also acts as a fabric softener and deodorizer.

Additional Information on the Blood Type Diet

Discover Your Blood Type

It is difficult to begin a diet based on blood type if you are not aware of your own type. In Europe, blood type is something almost everyone knows, but here in the United States, unless we need a transfusion, we can go our entire lives without knowing what blood type we are. Here are several simple ways to find out your type:

Donate blood. Not only are you providing a critical service to the community, but this is a free and simple way to find out what blood type you are. To find your local donation center, visit the American Red Cross website's Give Blood page (www.redcrossblood.org).

Purchase a blood-typing test kit at D'Adamo Personalized Nutrition (www.4yourtype.com), under "Books and Tests." The kit is inexpensive and simple to do in your own home.

Next time you visit your doctor for a blood workup, ask him or her to add blood type to the blood-draw protocol.

Secretor Status

In this book, we also address Secretor Status, tagging each recipe to indicate if it is appropriate for both Secretors and Non-Secretors. If you do not know your Secretor Status, you can purchase a Secretor Status Test Kit from D'Adamo Personalized Nutrition (www.4yourtype.com).

Center of Excellence in Generative Medicine

The Center of Excellence in Generative Medicine (COEGM) is a collaboration between Dr. Peter D'Adamo and the University of Bridgeport to create a frontiers-focused biomedical initiative without parallel in any other medical school. The COEGM combines patient care, clinical research, and hands-on teaching opportunities for students in UB's Health Sciences program. It is also home to Dr. Peter D'Adamo's clinical practice. For information and appointments for either private practice–patients or clinic-shift patients, please contact:

Center of Excellence in Generative Medicine
115 Broad Street
Bridgeport, CT 06604
(203) 366-0526
www.generativemedicine.org/

D'Adamo Personalized Nutrition®—North American Pharmacal, Inc.

For information on the Blood Type Diet, individualized supplements, and testing kits, please contact:
D'Adamo Personalized Nutrition
North American Pharmacal, Inc
213 Danbury Road
Wilton, CT 06897
International: (203) 761-0042
Toll-Free USA: (877) 226-8973
Fax: (203) 761-0043
www.4yourtype.com

www.dadamo.com—For All Things Peter D'Adamo

One of the longest running websites on the Internet, www.dadamo.com is the home page for the community of netizens who follow the work of Dr. Peter D'Adamo. This easy-to-navigate site is chockful of helpful tools, blogs, and one of the warmest, most welcoming chat forums to be found. Newbies are welcome to this moderated, family-friendly community.

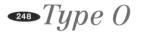

Products

Dr. D'Adamo's products used in this book and where to find them:

Protein Blend™ Powder—Type O

Dr. D'Adamo created a specific protein powder to benefit the individual needs of each blood type. The Type O powder has a high protein content based on rice protein and egg whites, and contains no sugar.

Protein Blend Powder can be purchased online at: www.4yourtype.com, simply click "Specialty Products" and scroll down to find "Bars and Shakes."

Unibar® Protein Bar

The Unibar® is the healthy snack you don't have to feel guilty about! Designed by Dr. D'Adamo for all blood types, including Secretors and Non-Secretors, the Unibar® is ideal as a meal replacement, clean-fuel workout bar, or nutritious snack for a burst of energy between meals.

Chocolate Cherry (15 grams of protein) and Blueberry Almond (13 grams of protein) Unibar®s can be purchased online at: www.4yourtype .com, simply click "Specialty Products" and scroll down to "Bars and Shakes."

Carob Extract™

This delicious, irresistible syrup made from the carob bean is *Beneficial* for all blood types for easing digestive discomfort as well as for coping with fatigue. It's so good that 1 teaspoon a day won't be enough! Use as a topping on crêpes, ice cream, muffins, and even cereals.

Carob Extract™ can be purchased online at: www.4yourtype.com, simply click "Specialty Products" and scroll down to find "Bars and Shakes."

Proberry 3™ Liquid

Developed for immune support, Proberry 3™ comes in both capsules and liquid, but after tasting the liquid you will be hooked! Drink it by the teaspoonful when you have a cold, or drizzle it in smoothies, mix into ice cream, or stir into tea for a tasty boost of antioxidants.

Proberry 3™ can be purchased online at: www.4yourtype.com, simply click "Right for All Types," then "Immune Support" and scroll down to find Proberry 3™ Liquid.

For a complete list of all products formulated by Dr. Peter J. D'Adamo, go to www.4yourtype.com.

SWAMI© Personalized Nutrition Software Program

Dr. D'Adamo developed the SWAMI software to harness the power of computers and artificial intelligence, using their tremendous precision and speed to help tailor unique one-of-a kind diets.

From its extensive knowledge base, SWAMI can evaluate more than 700 foods for more than 200 individual attributes (such as cholesterol level, gluten content, presence of antioxidants, etc.) to determine if that food is either a superfood or toxin for you. It provides a specific one of a kind diet in an easy-to-read, friendly format. For more information about SWAMI, you can go to www.4yourtype.com.

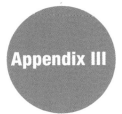
References

1. Bob's Red Mill. Bob's Red Mill Natural Foods. www.bobsredmill.com. Accessed May 2013.

2. D'Adamo, Peter J., and Whitney, Catherine. *Eat Right 4 Your Type*. New York: G. P. Putnam's Sons, 1996.

3. D'Adamo, Peter J., and Whitney, Catherine. *Live Right 4 Your Type*. New York: G. P. Putnam's Sons, 2001.

4. D'Adamo, Peter J., and Whitney, Catherine. *Blood Type O Food, Beverage, and Supplements Lists from Eat Right 4 Your Type*, New York: The Berkley Publishing Group, 2002.

5. "EWG's Shopper's Guide to Pesticides in Produce." Environmental Working Group, www.ewg.org, 2011.

6. "Food Labeling/Organic Foods," United States Department of Agriculture, www.usda.gov. Accessed May 2013.

7. "Healthy Child, Healthy World." www.healthychild.org. Accessed May 2013.

8. Mateljan, George. "The World's Healthiest Foods." www.whfoods.com. Accessed May 2013.

9. Nischan, Michel, and Goodbody, Mary. *Sustainably Delicious: Making the World a Better Place, One Recipe at a Time*. New York: Rodale Books, 2010.

Acknowledgments

PETER J. D'ADAMO

It is with great pleasure to share with the readers of *Eat Right 4 Your Type* and followers of my work on the Blood Type Diet and my continuing explorations in the area of personalized medicine the *Eat Right 4 Your Type Personalized Cookbook* series. There are many people I would like to thank, as this was a group effort.

My deep appreciation to Berkley Books, a division of Penguin Group (USA) Inc., as my longtime publisher; in particular, my editor, Denise Silvestro, whose personal belief in these cookbooks brought them from their original e-book format to where we are today; publisher, Leslie Gelbman; and Allison Janice, who coordinated the production efforts; Pam Barricklow, the managing editor; and the entire Berkley team who worked on these books. I would also like to thank my dedicated agent, Janis Vallely, whose encouragement, guidance, and tenacity have made this book possible.

A very special thanks to Kristin O'Connor, whose culinary skills combined with her depth of knowledge of and belief in the Blood Type Diet, have allowed us to develop delicious, nutritious recipes that are right for each type.

A special nod of appreciation for our team at North American Pharmacal and Drum Hill, who worked on these books as they were being developed, especially Bob Messineo, Wendy Simmons-Taylor, Ann Quasarano, John Alvord, Emily D'Adamo, and Angela Bergamini.

As always, I am grateful to my wife and partner, Martha Mosko D'Adamo, for her unwavering support and for the role she played in shepherding these books into existence; and to my two daughters, Claudia and Emily, who share a deep passion for this work and for a well-cooked meal.

A final thanks to the hundreds of thousands of readers and followers who have shared this journey with me. I am encouraged and fortified by your continuing dedication to your personal health and well-being, and I am humbled by your trust and commitment to this work.

KRISTIN O'CONNOR

I am so fortunate to have such a huge arena of support; I truly could not have done it without any of you.

First, of course is Dr. Peter D'Adamo, the science behind this effective diet. I will always respect your brilliant mind and interest in making this world a healthier place. To my mother, Susan O'Connor, for being the reason I had so much faith in this diet, teaching me how to cook, supporting my every move, and being there by my side while I tested all six hundred recipes! To my father, Kevin O'Connor, who sees more potential in me than anyone I've ever met, guided me in the basics of photography, and taught me to have the courage to put myself out there over and over again. To my brother, Dr. Ryan O'Connor, for valuing my accomplishments and always sharing in the joys of my success as if they were his own . . . and being a very willing recipe-testing guinea pig! To my grandparents Mike and Ellie DeMaio, thank you for being my cheerleaders, and providing encouragement and unconditional support.

A huge thank you to David Domedion who meticulously edited every recipe. Thank you to Chris Bierlein for his incredible talent, kind spirit, and generosity with shooting and editing our gorgeous cover photos. We were privileged to work with you.

Heather Rahilly, whose friendship kept me sane and whose intellect kept me in the race, thank you for being the most thorough attorney I could ask for! To my friends, who are all like family to me, for selflessly offering help in any way they could: Annie Gaffron, Mandy Geisler, Latha Chirunomula (along with Padma and Pushpavathi for teaching me the basics of South Indian cooking), Jennifer Eastes, Iwona Lacka, and the Metwallys.

Thank you to Tim Macklin for being my very patient mentor, and a great source of knowledge and encouragement. Thanks to Danielle Boccher, Scott Olnhausen, and the rest of my pals at Concentric! Special thanks to Dr. Peter Bongiorno and Dr. Pina LoGiudice for taking me under their wing when I was just a little fledgling cook wanting to make a difference.

Thank you to Kate Fitzpatrick and Ann Quasarano, whose dependability and efforts at getting our book out there in the public eye was very much appreciated. Thanks to Stephen Czick for his hours of editing and support, and Wendy Simmons-Taylor for all her patience with styling these books.

Thanks to Martha D'Adamo and the team at Drum Hill Publishing for giving me the opportunity to work on these cookbooks, which I very much love and believe in.

And finally, a very special thank you to Craig Anderson for taking a chance on me at the very beginning and opening the doors to my dreams.

About the Authors

PETER J. D'ADAMO

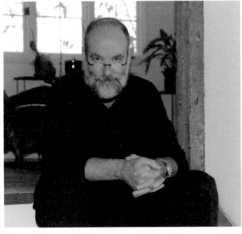

A second-generation naturopathic doctor, Dr. D'Adamo has been practicing naturopathic medicine for more than thirty years. Best known for his research on human blood groups and nutrition, Dr. D'Adamo is also a well-respected researcher in the field of natural products and a Distinguished Professor of Clinical Sciences at the University of Bridgeport. He is the founder and director of the Center of Excellence in Generative Medicine, a clinical, academic, and research institute, which also houses his private clinical practice located in a beautifully restored Victorian house on the campus of the University of Bridgeport overlooking the Long Island Sound. Dr. D'Adamo is the recipient of the 1990 AANP Physician of the Year Award for his role in the creation of the *Journal of Naturopathic Medicine*.

Dr. D'Adamo's series of books are *New York Times* bestsellers and Book-of-the-Month-Club® selections. He was named the "Most Intriguing Health Author of 1999," and his first book, *Eat Right 4 Your Type* was voted one of the "Ten Most Influential Health Books of All Time" by media industry analysts. *Publishers Weekly* called his third book, *Live Right 4 Your Type*, "A comprehensive and fascinating theory that has been meticulously researched." His books have been translated into sixty-five languages, and there are over seven million copies of his books worldwide.

KRISTIN O'CONNOR

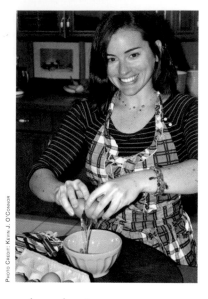

PHOTO CREDIT: KEVIN J. O'CONNOR

Kristin has made it her life's work to create food that is irresistibly tasty and healthy, a combination she hopes will inspire people to love good, healthy food and encourage them to make healthy eating a lifelong habit. In doing so, she created NourishThis.com—a website with recipes, articles, and tips on eating well and living green; volunteers for Healthy Child, Healthy World—a nonprofit that educates parents about nutritional and environmental issues affecting their children; and presented at the Kids Food Festival in New York City. She has worked for a Food Network and Cooking Channel production company as an associate producer on many of their shows, was an above-the-line catering chef for a lead actor on a major motion picture, and is now working as a private celebrity chef. Kristin continues to volunteer for nonprofit organizations that promote a healthy diet and environment, and hopes to continue her career as a cookbook author in the future.